The *Fast* Diabetes Solution

A Holistic Formula for Reversing Diabetes
and Living a Healthy, Happy Life

Suzanne Ridley

with Steve Eggleston

Address all inquiries to:

Email: suzanne@puranutrients.com

PuraNutrients.com

ISBN-13: 978-1984959119

ISBN-10: 1984959115

First Edition, March 2018

Editor: David Scott

Cover: Diren Yardimli

Interior Design: David Scott

Every attempt has been made to source properly all quotes.

Health Caution:

†Results may vary. Information and statements made are for education purposes and are not intended to replace the advice of your doctor. FDS does not dispense medical advice, prescribe, or diagnose illness. The views and nutritional advice expressed by FDS are not intended to be a substitute for conventional medical service. If you have a severe medical condition or health concern, see your physician.

ABOUT THE AUTHOR

I have been a pharmacist for over 40 years. Twenty years ago, due to my special interest in diet and health, I embarked on further study. Obtaining a post-graduate diploma in Clinical Nutrition, I opened my eyes to the powerful role played by diet and nutrients in our health, and how deficiencies in nutrients set us up for health problems later in life, including type 2 diabetes, obesity, and heart disease. When a friend introduced me to herbalism, I embraced it with open arms and became passionate about the natural, holistic side to health.

Despite my pharmacological background, I was struck with how many gaps herbalism filled in my knowledge and experience in helping patients with their health. I loved the way these herbs had their own special qualities to nurture ailments and address health issues in ways more subtle than drugs and with far fewer side effects. Armed with my Diplomas in Medical Herbalism and Clinical Nutrition and inspired by what I had learned, I felt better equipped to assist my clients and deal with their health needs.

You could say that I have developed a complementary approach to medicine, seeing the value in both schools of thought and appreciating the balance required in diet, exercise, and stress management in order to live a happy, healthy life. It is with this point of view that I approach solutions to one of the most pervasive and deadly epidemics of our time: type 2 diabetes.

Proudly brought to you by
Pura Nutrients

DEDICATION

In memory of my dear friend, Heather. A passionate believer in natural health, Heather opened my eyes to the vast benefits of herbal medicine.

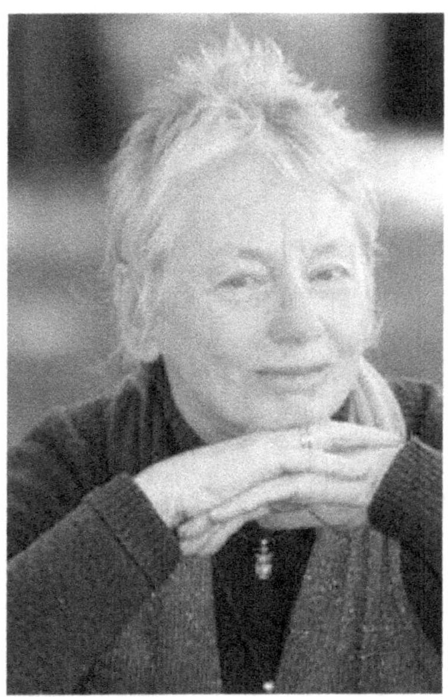

CONTENTS

"It is health that is real wealth and not pieces
of gold and silver."

~ Mahatma Gandhi

ACKNOWLEDGMENTS

I would like to thank my husband, Ray, for his enduring faith in me. His knowledge of Traditional Chinese Medicine adds another color to the palette.

My son, Patrick — his vision, persistence, and unbounded energy have made this book possible.

My teachers:

Denis Stewart of the Southern Cross Herbal School, an internationally recognized expert in Western Herbal Medicine, I will always be grateful for your infectious passion for herbs.

Dr. Robert Buist of The International Academy of Nutrition, a noted biochemist, you have taught me the value of nutrition and the invaluable role of nutrients in maintaining health and warding off illness.

To my many clients and customers, your health struggles have shown me the great need for information that will allow and compel you to play a positive and active role in your own health choices.

A special acknowledgement goes to:

– Professor Roy Taylor of Newcastle University of England, for your inspiring research in the face of initial opposition.

Suzanne Ridley

– Dr. Jason Fung, for your commendable work on obesity and type 2 diabetes, helping to bring the truth to the surface for all to see.

– Professor Jenny Brand-Miller of Sydney University, for your extensive research into the Glycemic Index.

And lastly, though certainly not least, a very special thank you to Steve Eggleston, whose guidance has transformed my message into this marvelous book you are about to read.

To all of you, I owe an unending debt of gratitude hopefully repaid, in some small part, by this little but powerful book.

PREFACE
A Few Words from Suzanne

No one can dispute the many benefits of modern medicine and pharmaceutical drugs in treating type 2 diabetes. For a large part of my career as a pharmacist, I have been on the front lines with these medications, entrenched in the drug-based model of treating patients by treating ailments. The primary focus has been on treatment, not prevention. Under the current system, there is little tolerance for advocating a preventive model for health care, and few doctors advise on it (though the number is increasing every year).

For me, seeing what I've seen, this pill-oriented approach to patient care leaves far too many questions unanswered, and nowhere is it more evident in the traditional treatment of type 2 diabetes. Sadly, the misguided emphasis on drugs as a primary (and often only) treatment has ignored the causes and natural solutions to this unnecessarily debilitating and life-threatening illness.

So many clients who complain to me about fatigue, repeated infections, or struggling with their weight could not find acceptable answers in the traditional approach. There were no drugs that would effectively combat their constellation of problems. Witnessing this first-hand is what launched me on my personal journey to seek out the other modalities desperately needed to fill the gaps. That is where the holistic, health-based systems of nutrition, herbalism, and stress management truly shine — filling those gaps and showing their many strengths.

I have been fortunate in my life to have had many teachers, mentors, and friends to assist me in this journey, and I am proud to offer my readers **The *Fast* Diabetes Solution**™.

Introduction

In the scary world of type 2 diabetes, there are only two things that matter: Information and Action. So after a few questions to start us off, that's how we'll approach the solution.

A Few Questions

I ask you:

Have you been battling (over-consuming) cookies, crisps, chips, puddings, soda, candy bars, sweets, processed foods, refined sugar, and fast food for as long as you can remember?

Are you so exhausted by the time you do the school runs, finish work, wash clothes, clean house, make meals, and attend to everyone else's needs — that you're too tired to exercise your own body or tend to yourself?

Has negative energy — from the news, politics, and modern-day rat race — taken over your life?

Are you so stressed you can barely sleep at night?

Have you lost your figure, energy, and optimism for a happy and healthy life after retirement?

Have you been compensating by eating fast food and sugar-laden packaged snacks, then washing them down with soda or juice?

Suzanne Ridley

Do you find yourself waiting in line at the local pharmacy so often they know your first name — so often that taking prescribed pills has replaced eating a healthy diet, exercising, and managing your stressors?

Are you feeling overwhelmed — not knowing how to start dropping excess fat, losing weight and getting your health back on track?

Do you have type 2 diabetes or have you "life-styled" your way into pre-diabetes or obesity?

All of that can and will change by reading this book. Here you will find a **Fast** solution to reversing your diabetes. But by **Fast**, I do not mean speedy solutions that are done and finished in the blink of an eye.

Fast in my book combines elements that are speedy — fasting and Tabata work at lightning speed — with elements that last a lifetime — a healthy diet, exercise, and stress management.

That said, don't get me wrong. The health benefits you will feel will indeed be **Fast**. For many, following the methods urged in this book their type 2 diabetes have been reversed within weeks.

Yet whether it takes you weeks or months to reach the results you need, it will be a relatively fast and enjoyable recovery well worth the effort you undertake.

Compared to the outdated mainstream mantra that "type 2 diabetes is a progressive disease you'll have for life," you will start to experience positive results very quickly.

Soon, with head held high, you will walk past the unfortunate type 2 diabetic who remains shackled to a "life sentence" of heart disease, lower limb amputations, blindness and premature death.

As you do, you'll realize the *Fast* and life-changing progress you have made.

Now, please walk over to the mirror and take a deep, long look at what you see. Then pull out your mobile phone and snap a photo of your current figure, so you'll be able to compare and contrast your body's transformation, say goodbye, and smile.

Yes, you will say goodbye to the former diabetic, pre-diabetic and/or obese you ("self, it was good to know you"), and congratulations to your new diabetes-free, thin, healthy, and stress-free self ("self, it is wonderful to make your acquaintance!").

But before I go any further, let me congratulate you, the reader, for taking this first crucial step towards living a healthy, diabetes-free lifestyle. Finding this book and reading this far is the first step toward your transformation.

Now, with introductions out of the way, let me anticipate your first question: How can simply reading a book reverse my diabetes, much less make me healthy for life?

The obvious answer is: it won't. It will take more than that. Sorry. Because you are part of the problem, you must become part of the solution. But, let me repeat what you already know: all solutions require a first step in the journey.

Suzanne Ridley

Of course, reading this book is not only your first step; it's also your most important step. Because with this one important step (a few hours on the couch or in bed reading for a few nights), your life will experience a domino effect. The end result will be a diabetes-free, healthy lifestyle for life.

Initially, you may feel doubt. Like so many other big challenges in life, at the outset, there's the grip of pessimism and the fear of failure. Or just the thought of the hassle or the belief that it won't work anyway, so why bother. Everyone goes through it, and if you let yourself, you'll find a gazillion reasons why you shouldn't even bother trying.

For starters, maybe you've tried umpteen types of approaches and failed — the latest fad diet, the new celebrity workout, another miracle diet pill. Some maybe even worked for a moment before fading away.

Now, against that history, I'm just someone else — in this case, not even a celebrity — who is asking you to begin another lonely journey which will probably fail once again.

Banish those thoughts. I won't ask you to do it alone. I will arm you with what you need to know to both reverse your diabetes and create a healthy lifestyle going forward. In fact, let me take this opportunity to introduce you to your team — you've known many of them for years.

Here they are: your insulin, your muscles, your metabolism, your circadian rhythm, your cellular intelligence, your gut, your discerning mind, healthy food, herbs, spices, exercise, meditation, sleep, and of course your doctor — we're all going to do this together.

Whoa! Slow down, you say. You're already talking team and I haven't even given you the *Fast* solution. Please be patient, I will, I'll get right to that.

But before I do, I'm going to do something unusual. I'm going to break the cardinal rule of story-telling. I'm going to reveal to you the ending of the story at the beginning. Why? To motivate you to reach the end.

You have now arrived at a fork-in-the-road where your storyline will go one of two ways: One is a sad and dark path to a shortened life full of suffering and heavy, pill-driven medical costs. The other — well, I'm going to let you decide what that is based on the solution provided in this book.

But, I assure you that most of you can be completely free of diabetes in the not too distance future, and all of you who follow my guidelines will live much healthier and happier lives.

That said, when you put this book down and surf the internet or go out into the world, you will be bombarded with a storm of negativity and pessimism. Many doctors and dieticians will tell you that type 2 diabetes is a chronic, progressive disease that cannot be cured or reversed — meaning, you're stuck with it for the rest of your life, and it's only going to get worse.

In my opinion, for most of you, that's utter and total nonsense. And if you buy it, you'll fall victim to a self-fulfilling prophecy based on outdated and outright false information. But how can that be, you ask? It's simple. Even in medicine, old ways die hard.

Historically, the mainstream medical fraternity, of which I've been a member for 40+ years, has used a drug-based approach to treating people who have already contracted diabetes. This approach is slowly being replaced by preventive methods — diet, exercise, and stress control — that also provide a non-drug treatment solution.

So let's get to the nitty-gritty. Reversing type 2 diabetes is directly linked to two things: removing your insulin resistance, and ridding your body of the internal body fat that's killing you.

This book will give you **Fast** solutions to both: by showing you how to dissolve your internal fat, thereby freeing your pancreas and liver to be healthy, reducing insulin resistance and chronic inflammation — all of which send your body into a downward diabetes spiral, pushing you closer to the emergency room each and every day.

But that's not all this book will do. As you take this first step, we want you to be inspired. We want you to start building confidence and momentum. To start embracing good spirits and positive energy about the journey ahead and the profound changes that are about to unfold in your life.

Ready to get started? Ready to step outside of your box? To expand your comfort zone and fully transform into the person that you are already becoming?

Ready to achieve your health goals? To banish your negative mindset? To change your history of eating unhealthy foods? To exercise and manage your stress and change your lifestyle for the better?

Ready to reverse your type 2 diabetes — forever?

Fantastic. Let's take this journey together and achieve a sustaining, ongoing diabetes-free lifestyle of health and happiness.

Let's go. You can do it!

Action:

At the end of each chapter, including this one, we will ask you to take action, calling upon the age-old wisdom: "success is bias to action."

As you go, also put aside time each day to summarize what you've learned and what you plan to do about it. We will guide you, but keep this in mind as you curate your motivation: the healthy you and a diabetes-free lifestyle is waiting for you at *The End.*

Start by writing your commitment to finishing this book. Jot down some times in the next week or two you know you have free (or can make free) to complete this book. An hour or two each or every other day should see you through the book and onto your new diabetes-free lifestyle before you know it.

Suzanne Ridley

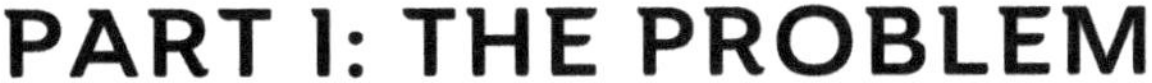

PART I: THE PROBLEM

Chapter 1
THE SILENT EPIDEMIC

"Don't dig your grave with your own knife and
fork."

– Old English Proverb

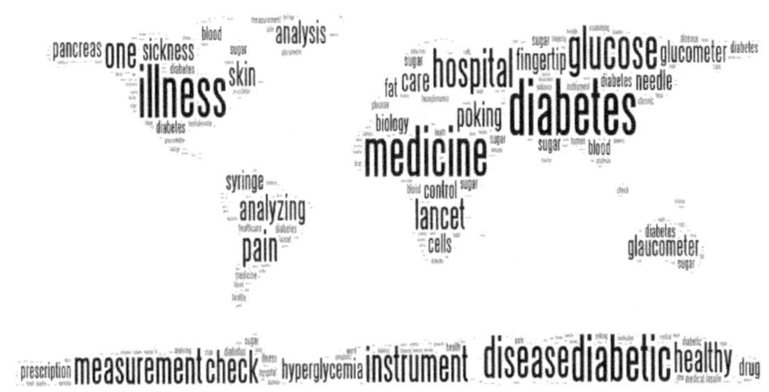

Information

Let's start with something you may already know,
because it bears emphasis from the outset: **YOU ARE
NOT ALONE**.

It's hard to imagine, but there are over 400 million
type 2 diabetics on the planet and in the U.S. alone
there are over 115 million Americans who are diabetic
or pre-diabetic, with some estimates as high as 150
million. A staggering 1.4 million Americans are
diagnosed with diabetes every year. Nearly seven

million people are diabetic but haven't been diagnosed. Put another way, over half of all Americans over 20 years of age are diabetic or pre-diabetic! Sadly, of that group, 73,000 will suffer "lower-limb amputations" with 60% of all such amputations occurring in diagnosed diabetics.

Generally speaking, these same devastating statistics hold equally true in Europe, Australia, and China. Yes, the Chinese have the largest diabetes epidemic in the world. As a result, healthcare practitioners worldwide are deeply concerned about the current state of human beings with diabetes. In America, the diabetes community presents the largest challenge in U.S. history to the country's sprawling health care system. The American Diabetes Association estimates the cost of addressing this pernicious disease to be in the hundreds of billions of dollars, every year!

To put the scope of the epidemic in perspective historically, consider these facts. In all of World War I, 41 million suffered death or injury. In World War II, that number leaped to 50 to 80 million, plus casualties, given the vastly greater firepower available. This figure includes the deaths and injured from both atom bombs, in all countries. The Black Plague of the 14th Century killed 100 million. And AIDS, since its inception, has killed upward of 70 million.

The sad truth for type 2 diabetics, however, is that much of this could be avoided by proper diet, exercise, and stress management. If we look back only as far as the 1950s, diabetes was uncommon. Most people didn't know a diabetic. A rounded meal of meat and three veggies was the norm, with a special dessert once or twice a week.

A more healthy diet, combined with natural, regular exercise caused people to be thinner. In the 1950s, 10% of a much smaller U.S. population was considered obese. Today that number has ballooned to 35% or one in three Americans, adding up to well over 110 million Americans. But it's not like everyone in the old days was working out at the gym or riding their lifecycles into oblivion, either. In America, through fitness guru Jack LaLanne's popular TV show that ran in the 1950s, the first health clubs with diverse exercise machines did not open until the early 1970s.

Before the advent of health clubs, exercise came from playing at the park, taking long walks, hiking nature's trails, gardening, housework, and sports, combined with whatever calories were burned off at work. Many people lived conservatively, on their budgets. The billions of dollars of tempting credit cards — often leading to unhealthy indulgences and debt-based stress — did not exist. Nor were supermarkets packed to the brim with unhealthy processed food, refined sugar, soda pop, and carbohydrate-dense junk food.

But there's more to the old ways. A daily eating habit that is commonplace today once was rare: snacking between meals. Though sugar snack ads started running on TV in the 1950s, seeking to reach the new demographic, teenagers, it wasn't until the 1970s that Big Food companies really ramped up their TV ad game, with millions of dollars being spent on slick spots promoting sugar-coated cereal to start the day, sweet and salty snacks between every meal (there's a whole aisle in the grocery store for that now), and loads of sugary-sweet desserts for after dinner or before bedtime.

But as profits soared for Big Food, especially with the addition of high fructose corn syrup (HFCS) to sweeten the allure of many processed foods and snacks, people went from eating three times a day to eating six, seven, even eight times a day, often consuming large helpings of highly-processed snacks, junk food, and fast foods laden with processed sugar, bad carbs, reams of preservatives, lots of table salt, and HFCS.

Of course, much research into the role played by carbohydrates in raising blood sugar had not yet been conducted, so some of this phenomenon was borne of ignorance. As a result, at this stage mainstream medicine was mostly in the dark about how the newly-available carbohydrates — processed foods and snacks — were contributing to the massive spiking of insulin in our collective pancreases, which resulted in a tidal wave of increased blood glucose in our societal blood.

Even though William Banting's 1863 book, Letter on Corpulence, revealed a very likely link between weight loss and carbohydrate restriction, and secretive 1960s tests at Harvard fingered carbohydrates, it wasn't until the early 1980s when American nutrition professor Dr. David Jenkins created the Glycemic Index (or GI) that we gained scientific evidence. The GI is a system that looks at the rate at which carbohydrates are converted to glucose in the blood. High glycemic carbs — high-GI carbs — are those that quickly break down into glucose to provide the body energy, thereby increasing your blood glucose levels and spiking your insulin production.

Low GI is the opposite of high GI. Low-GI carbs are those that break down slowly into glucose, causing a moderate glucose increase and moderate insulin response, causing the body to find energy burning fats instead. In her *Low GI Handbook: The New Glucose Revolution Guide to the Long-Term Health Benefits of Low GI,* Professor Jenny Brand-Miller of Sydney University describes low-GI carbs as "Tricklers" and high-GI carbs as "Gushers". It's a good way to visualize the process in your mind every time you think of reaching for a donut or bagel. When you bite into the donut, your pancreas yells "charge." In moments insulin is secreting like gangbusters into your blood to address the rising blood glucose.

At first, Western doctors were so confounded with the rise in diabetes, obesity, and heart disease (which is used interchangeably with cardiovascular disease, meaning clogged or blocked arteries) that they couldn't put a finger on it. Unable to pinpoint why so many patients were presenting as pre-diabetic, diabetic and obese, they ascribed it generally to "Metabolic Syndrome," a label created to describe the constellation of symptoms.

"Metabolic Syndrome" is a cluster of the most dangerous heart attack risk factors: diabetes and pre-diabetes, abdominal obesity, high cholesterol and high blood pressure. The International Diabetes Federation (IDF) worldwide definition of the Metabolic Syndrome provides physicians with the tools to quickly identify those at risk and also to compare the impact across nations and ethnic groups.

As time passed, it became more and more evident that "Metabolic Syndrome" was not going away; instead it was getting worse. At the 76th Scientific Session of the American Diabetes Association in New Orleans in 2016, ADA President Desmond Schatz, MD, described the diabetes trend as "alarming" and "like a wildfire raging through this country and across the globe," then, in utter amazement, asked the simple and profound rhetorical question: "[I]s anyone really paying attention?"

If you had to put a word on it, you might say that the modern world has fallen victim to *overindulgence* — eating too much of the wrong things too often, sneaking sugary and salty snacks between every meal, devouring too much fast food, and loading up on bad carbs while blind to the resulting high blood glucose and insulin spike. Blind, in particular, to the slippery slope to type 2 diabetes, pre-diabetes, and obesity — to which these all have led.

Looking at it today, it is quite clear that for decades we have been sold the wrong story. Because of this, as Yuval Noah Harari recently observed in his bestselling novel, *Homo Deus, A Brief History of Tomorrow*: "In 2012 about 5.6 million people died throughout the world; 620,000 of them died due to human violence (war killed 120,000 people, and crime killed another 500,000). In contrast, 800,000 committed suicide, and 1.5 million died of diabetes. **Sugar is now more dangerous than gunpowder**." [Emphasis added]

You can help reverse this trend beginning right now, so again grab your pen and put it to work.

Action

List out in detail what you normally eat each day of the week, including all meals and snacks as well as the amounts or portion sizes. Be stone cold honest, because your health and happiness depend on it.

Monday

Tuesday

Wednesday

Thursday

Friday

Saturday

Sunday

A friendly reminder. Please go back after a day or two and make sure you didn't leave anything out. When you prepare your *Fast* Diabetes-Free Lifestyle Plan at the end of Part III of the book, cross-reference to these answers to see just how far you have come.

Chapter 2
DIABETES AND HOW IT WORKS

"Ignorance is bliss, but not for long."

– Suzanne Ridley

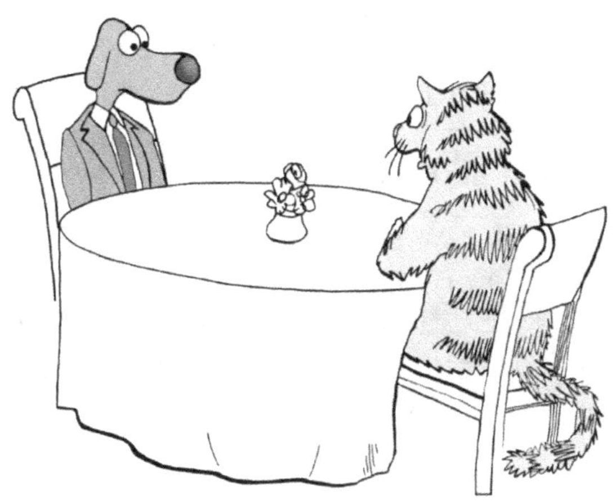

Information

To understand how diabetes works, and what can go wrong when it takes hold, let's look at how our body functions.

First, blood glucose is controlled by two hormones — insulin and glucagon. Both are secreted by the pancreas. When we eat, our blood glucose rises, and this signals our pancreas to release insulin.

Insulin then transports our increased blood glucose to our cells, where it is either used right away as energy (burned you might say) or stored as glycogen to be later converted to glucose and released into the bloodstream when energy is required. As glucose is removed from our blood, our blood insulin level drops correspondingly.

About four to six hours later, glucagon is released from the pancreas, whereby the stored glycogen is turned into glucose and released into the bloodstream to be used as energy. As a result, these two pancreatic hormones — insulin and glucagon — work together in a negative feedback system to regulate blood-sugar levels.

Many people don't understand this process or know the difference between type 1 and type 2 diabetes, much less conditions such as pre-diabetes or gestational diabetes. Even some people diagnosed with diabetes don't know the difference.

But knowing the difference matters, especially when it comes to reversing diabetes and adopting a healthy lifestyle solution. So let's take a look at the different incarnations of diabetes.

Type 2 Diabetes

Type 2 diabetes was once called mature onset diabetes, because it was most often associated with the elderly. This is no longer the case. The incidence of type 2 diabetes in younger people is increasing every year, with the youngest recorded diabetic in America being three years old.

Type 2 diabetes takes hold when the body's insulin resistance is so strong it cannot respond properly to the very insulin it produces, i.e., when it cannot transport the glucose from the blood to be stored in muscle, liver, and other cells of the body.

As a consequence, these cells are brimming with glucose as there is no more room. Insulin, being a storage hormone, then transports the excess glucose in the blood to be stored as fat — and for fat, the body allows plenty of room. We see it in our spare tires, love handles, paunch, gut or whatever you want to call it.

Unfortunately, this fat is also laid down — stored — deep in the abdominal cavity in and around our vital organs. What develops are fatty vital organs — a fatty liver, a fatty pancreas, etc. — that are weighted down and don't work efficiently and effectively.

The pancreas does not give up easily, however, so it struggles to produce more insulin. Not that it's tired or burned out. It's not that. Rather, it's just clogged with fat and must work extra hard to do its job (imagine wearing too many coats or jumpers).

As will be explained in later chapters, through **The *Fast* Diabetes-Free Lifestyle**, which combines fasting, healthy diet, exercise and stress management, type 2 diabetes is not only managed but often reversed forever as part of a Diabetes-Free Lifestyle Plan that will make you happier and healthier than you've been in years.

Type 1 Diabetes

Type 1 diabetes means the pancreas is not properly functioning, i.e., little or no insulin is being produced. This bit of information reminds us that little or no insulin is not the goal. That can be deadly.

Insulin itself is a hormone produced in the pancreas of a healthy body by beta cells. Once produced, the insulin hormone enters the bloodstream where it regulates the volume of glucose in your blood, moving it throughout the body to be used as fuel or stored as fat.

Because of the essential role played by the insulin hormone, the type 1 diabetic is always reliant on insulin injections. Without insulin, the glucose in the bloodstream cannot be moved into the cells and remains in the blood. The body is literally starving for energy. Medical experts view this condition as an autoimmune reaction whereby the body's immune system attacks and destroys the beta cells in the pancreas, thus rendering them unable to produce the insulin hormone that's needed for health.

According to the American Society for Metabolic and Bariatric Surgery, only 5% of diabetics are type 1. Eating well and making smart lifestyle choices helps to ward off further complications, but this particular illness does not result from poor dietary or lifestyle choices. Indeed, if you are someone with type 1 diabetes, rapid weight loss may be considered both undesirable and dangerous.

That important point reminds us of a crucial caveat: when considering the *Fast* options presented by this book, be sure to consult with your physician.

Gestational Diabetes

Gestational diabetes sometimes appears during pregnancy and is treated with insulin. It is thought to result from insulin resistance brought about by a rash of hormones secreted by a pregnant woman's placenta, which in turn makes the mother's insulin ineffective. Unfortunately, having gestational diabetes makes both mother and child more prone to developing type 2 diabetes later in life.

Though smart food choices combined with a well-balanced diet are essential to the health of a gestational diabetic, and to any mother carrying child, again this is not the time for the kind of fasting that works so well to reverse type 2 diabetes. As with type 1 diabetics, if you are a gestational diabetic, fasting is never suitable as a treatment option. Instead you are urged to stick to the smart food choices and healthy lifestyle otherwise suggested by this book, and of course to always consult your physician.

Pre-Diabetes

Pre-diabetes precedes diabetes, as denoted by the prefix. When an indication of pre-diabetes arrives, that means your insulin resistance is increasing and your blood-sugar levels are climbing higher — beyond what is considered normal and healthy — but not high enough for a full-on diagnosis of type 2 diabetes.

In other words, from a health point-of-view, you are moving in the wrong direction and need to make adjustments fast in order to avoid the diabetic cliff.

And don't be fooled. Your pre-diabetic state may last for ten or more years as your body's cells become more resistant to the effects of insulin and your internal fat increases gradually like a slow-moving snowball.

People with pre-diabetes face a serious increase in the risk that they will eventually develop type 2 diabetes and be stricken with cardiovascular disease, which can lead to a heart attack or stroke. Fortunately for you, since type 2 diabetes can be reversed, that means you don't have to saddle yourself with a full-on type 2 diabetes diagnosis in the first place. Like the disease itself, your pre-diabetic symptoms can be permanently reversed, never to return.

All it takes is information, action, and the willpower gained from reading a simple little book.

Action

If you have been diagnosed with diabetes or pre-diabetes, make a note of the time, date, and place of the diagnosis (ideally you will obtain these records and learn exactly what you have).

Make a list of all medications (pharmaceutical and other) you have taken and/or are taking to treat your diabetes or pre-diabetes, noting the effectiveness and side-effects of each.

Write out the extent to which your physician has advised you on the role played in diabetes by diet, exercise and stress management, as opposed to or in addition to taking pharmaceutically-prescribed medications.

All of the above will likely demonstrate how reliant you have become on medications to treat a problem, rather than solutions to reverse or prevent the problem in the first place.

Chapter 3
THE MYTHS

"The great enemy of the truth is very often not the lie, deliberate, contrived and dishonest, but the myth, persistent, persuasive and unrealistic."

– John F. Kennedy

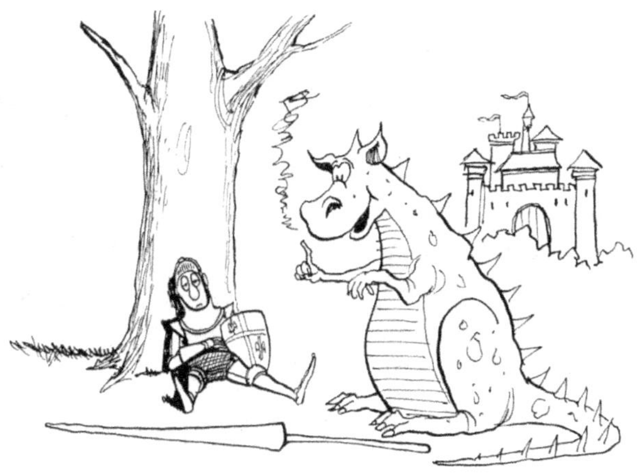

"We didn't have a nutritious breakfast,
did we?"

Information

In many fields of human endeavor, myths stand in the way of progress. In medicine, they mislead the suffering person and obscure the availability of a cure or better treatment to disease.

A myth, of course, can be many things. On the warm and fuzzy side, it can be ancient lore about a mythological Avalon King, or a popular tale like Herman Melville's *Moby Dick*, the battle of the great white whale. But when it comes to science, and in particular diabetes, the matter of myths takes a serious turn.

A scientific myth entails exaggeration, half-truth, or sometimes pure fanciful fiction that may undermine the Hippocratic Oath: "do no harm." Here are some myths about diabetes that may shock you.

Myth #1: Type 2 diabetes is an irreversible and progressive illness

Myth #1 Busted: Type 2 diabetes is reversible

The notion that diabetes as an illness cannot be reversed — that pre-diabetics and type 2 diabetics might as well toss in the towel — is at least an exaggeration, maybe even half-truth and, probably, 100% rubbish.

Embracing Myth #1 for years, the medical establishment has thrown mountains of pills at type 2 diabetes, the next regimen purportedly improving over the last and all effective in their own limited way, but none treating the underlying cause of the illness. Managed in this way, the diabetic patient is truly experiencing an irreversible and progressive illness, thereby making the myth self-fulfilling.

By now the ineffectiveness of throwing pills at type 2 diabetes as the sole treatment plan should, in my opinion, be evident. Ignoring billions of dollars in pills, cardiovascular disease holds strong as the number one cause of death for type 2 diabetics, accounting for a bone-chilling two-thirds of all deaths.

Who wants to be pill-popping all day while embarrassed to don a swimsuit at the beach due to an expanding, bulging waistline? Yet, if things continue in the direction they are headed, the forecast is gloomy: despite prescribing more meds than ever to control blood glucose levels and high blood pressure, the same medical fraternity predicts that many diabetic patients will end up injecting insulin and eventually succumbing to a cardiovascular episode such as a stroke or a heart attack.

To debunk the old pill-popping view, one can skip straight to the recent work of world-renowned Professor of Medicine & Metabolism at Newcastle University, Dr. Roy Taylor. His much vaunted 2016 study, published in Diabetes Care, reconfirms his ground-breaking 2011 study by concluding that 10-year diabetics can reverse or vastly improve their diabetes simply by honoring a regimen of 800 calories per day. Not to mention, Chinese herbalists have been preventing diabetes for years.

Indeed, Myth #1 is not only unabashedly wrong, it's leading us like lemmings over the proverbial diabetic cliff — fostering a pandemic of newly diagnosed diabetics despite the swell of new drugs being thrown at diabetes.

Uncloaking Myth #1 to mainstream medicine is of utmost importance. And that can begin with you.

Myth #2: I can eat what I want because I exercise regularly

Myth #2 Busted: Regular exercise is not enough

If anyone ever blamed exercise — or lack of it — as the primary culprit of type 2 diabetes, pre-diabetes, obesity, and cardiovascular disease, you'd think the accuser might be a gunslinger from the soda pop industry. And guess what, the soda pop industry has commissioned a study that does exactly that. While I'm not surprised, I am astounded at the chutzpah.

But before we discuss the Soda Pop Study, let's look at the battle of videos that led to it. The opening salvo was fired by British pharmacist Niraj Naik, who frightened soda pop drinkers by releasing a shocking infographic showing what happens to the human body one hour after a can of Coke or Diet Coke is consumed.

Coke's scientists counterpunched, pinning the primary blame for obesity on laziness, i.e., lack of exercise, citing to compelling evidence on the importance of exercise. And of course, they were right: exercise is important. But it is far from the most important factor in the development of type 2 diabetes and by no means should you down a liter of Coke because you plan to run a mile afterward.

That's not the whole story. The rest of the story comes from *The New York Times. The Times* dug deeper, and in an article entitled "Coca-Cola Funds Scientists Who Shift Blame for Obesity Away From Bad Diets," reported that a soft drink-friendly group by the name of Global Energy Balance Network partially financed and supported the lack-of exercise study.

In the real world, an excellent example of the tension between processed food, sugar and exercise played out on an Australian TV show known as *Catalyst*. In *Catalyst*, airing August 2016, a young, very fit gymnast and a middle-aged man were both fed high-carb meals and then measured for the effect of the carbs on their insulin levels. The presumption was that both bodies, despite their vast differences, would quickly break down their blood glucose with a contrasting spike in insulin production from the pancreas (little from the gymnast, a lot from the older man).

The results were astonishing: the young gymnast required more than double the amount of insulin to deal with his meals than the middle-aged man. Closer analysis of their diets revealed the underlying reason: The gymnast's diet consisted largely of junk food, i.e., left-over pizza for breakfast, hamburger and fries for lunch, and take-away for dinner — a diet consisting largely of high-GI (high glycemic) carbs.

Because he had been suffering from chronic allergies, the middle-aged man had long ago adopted a diet based on vegetables, good quality protein (somewhat of a Mediterranean diet), and exercise, though he certainly was no gymnast. In only decent shape on the outside due to his age, on the inside he was in much better condition than his younger, fitter counterpart. In other words, despite his aging outside appearance, on the inside he was fit-as-a-fiddle.

The solution for the gymnast was to have a major overhaul of his eating patterns. He knew it had to be done, but expressed concerns about whether he would like the taste of healthy foods. During his first week of low-GI carbs, as his body replaced junk food with loads of vegetables and fruit, his complaints were so rancorous the audience felt he might quit. Good theatre, but he didn't. He hung tight.

By week two, he was not only adjusting, he was joking about his sniveling and whining the previous week. Weeks three and four saw him enjoying his new food with a vigorous commitment to continue. In just one month, his body showed vast improvements, needing less than half the insulin than it previously needed to process the same meal. In other words, his insulin resistance had been dramatically reduced.

Poor diet, not exercise, had proven to be the primary factor in triggering insulin resistance, despite the crucial role played by exercise in leading a diabetes-free lifestyle.

Myth #3: Follow the traditional Food Guide Pyramid for optimum health

Myth #3 Busted: Yeah, follow it if you want to get fat

Everyone in America, and many people throughout the world, know about the hallowed Food Guide Pyramid. They see it on cereal boxes, bread wrappers, meat packages, egg cartons, and bags of pasta and nuts, as well as elementary school bulletin boards and university textbooks. For decades, it has been deemed the "Holy Grail" of U.S. dietary standards.

Could it be wrong? Yes. Dr. Walter Willet, a leading American nutrition researcher and Chairman of the

Nutrition Department at Harvard University, writes earnestly that it is. His new book, *Eat, Drink, and Be Healthy: The Harvard Medical School Guide to Healthy Eating*, postulates that the Food Pyramid goes astray, enlarging waistlines and harming health from diabetes to obesity.

The Food Pyramid advises the consumption per day of six to eleven servings of bread, cereal, rice, and pasta; two to three servings of meat, poultry, fish, dry beans, eggs, and nuts; and sparing consumption of fats, oils, and sweets. Sounds and feels pretty right on, you might say. And you should. You have been indoctrinated to think this way your whole life.

What then is wrong with a diet based on the Food Pyramid? To begin with, the Pyramid does not reflect the latest nutritional research. Dr. Willett observes as follows:

> "The thing to keep in mind about the USDA Pyramid is that it comes from the Department of Agriculture, the agency responsible for promoting American agriculture, not from agencies established to monitor and protect our health, like the Department of Health and Human Services, or the National Institutes of Health, or the Institute of Medicine.
>
> ... And there's the root of the problem — what's good for some agricultural interests isn't necessarily good for the people who eat their products... Serving two masters is tricky business, especially when one of them includes persuasive and well-connected representatives

of the formidable meat, dairy, and sugar industries.

... The end result of their tug-of-war is a set of positive, feel-good, all-inclusive recommendations that completely distort what could be the single most important tool for improving your health and the health of the nation... At best, the USDA Pyramid offers indecisive, scientifically unfounded advice on an absolutely vital topic — what to eat. At worst, the misinformation it offers contributes to obesity, poor health, and unnecessarily early death."

The misguided U.S. Food Pyramid was adopted as the law of the land in 1992, putting carbohydrates prominently at the base of the pyramid as foods to eat. However, the latest research — indeed, even substantial historical research — demonstrates that the Food Pyramid diet encourages excessive consumption of carbohydrates, both good and bad.

In so doing, it lumps mono-saturates, saturated fats, omega-3 fatty acids, omega-6 fatty acids, and trans-fatty acids all together. Not to mention, it fails to differentiate between sugars — sugar from fresh fruit and vegetables versus processed white sugar and high fructose corn syrup — despite the dramatic differences between them on insulin production and resistance.

Unfortunately, this single failure has contributed substantially — in falsely influencing the medical community, consumers, and policymakers — to the epidemic in dietary health from which the world suffers today. So yeah, be assured that if you keep eating as the Food Pyramid dictates, you will soon start to look like the Food Pyramid as your body slowly builds toward a wide-waisted life of diabetes, obesity and heart disease.

Myth #4: Fat causes heart disease

Myth #4 Busted: Fat is back

I have vivid memories of watching my sister making an omelet, separating the egg whites from the yokes and discarding the yokes in the bin before frying what remained with a tiny bit of water. Such was the obsession of much of society with fat avoidance. And guess what, there's a reason for that.

Beginning in the 1960s, fat was blamed for heart disease. By 1977, a low-fat diet was recommended to all Americans. This was a pivotal time, ushering in the modern era of chronic low-grade inflammation, obesity, cardiovascular disease and, you guessed it, diabetes, as we were throwing out butter and replacing it with margarine.

Margarine, unfortunately, is made from highly-processed vegetable oils that contain pro-inflammatory omega 6 fatty acids making them solid by adding trans-fatty acids. A double whammy. What a disaster!

Despite there being no evidence that saturated fat causes heart disease, this myth has been perpetuated persistently and proven very difficult to debunk. Several examples — the Polynesian Diet, the French Paradox, and the Greek Paradox — eloquently make the point.

Polynesians have reported remarkably low incidence of heart disease despite consuming for centuries diets heavily laden in saturated fat from coconuts (which make up 63% of their diets). If saturated fat were the true culprit, these statistics would need explaining. When scientists looked deeper, what they found is that the Polynesian diet was also persistently low in sugar and processed foods (the real culprits).

Showing allegiance to their own culinary culture, the French have long ignored the low-fat advice, continuing to cook with whole butter and whole cream. Amazingly, their levels of cardiovascular disease and obesity have not soared — instead, remaining constantly low. Befuddled by this fact, medical experts considered it a freak phenomenon and termed it "The French Paradox". So convinced were the experts that high fat was not the path to follow to reduce heart disease, that they attributed the result to the consumption of red wine.

Enter the Greeks, whose diet we could just as easily describe as the "Greek Paradox." The Greeks — with their Mediterranean diet full of antioxidant vegetables and lashings of olive oil, balsamic vinegar, and lemons — also continued to enjoy good health despite eating a traditional mix of foods high in fat.

By digging deeper, we now see how misguided dietary policy can also have a domino effect. Because fat tastes good, when it was removed from processed foods they lost the corresponding layer of good taste and yummy flavor that came with fat. To put taste and flavor back into the food, processed food makers turned to cheap processed sugar and cheaper HFCS.

The domino effect of adding processed sugar and HFCS to virtually all boxed and canned foods — thus making cardboard tasty — was to dramatically increase their proportion of bad carb intake. And guess what? Bingo! People started getting fatter and fatter as the fast-food franchises mushroomed and cardiovascular disease, obesity, and type 2 diabetes surged to epidemic numbers.

Unfortunately, few questioned the validity of this path and those important studies abdicating the doctrine of fat reduction were ignored.

Are you really saying eat more fat? You must be kidding. No, I am not. By eating the right mix of fat, the body gets healthier and fights back diabetic conditions. Fat is back on the menu, and guess what? It tastes good. But which fats am I referring to? In other words, what are the right fats?

To answer these questions, let's look more closely at different types of fat, as fat is one of the three macronutrients present in foods and is essential for survival.

The main fats can be categorized as follows: (1) saturated fats, (2) monounsaturated fats, and (3) omega-3 and omega-6 essential fatty acids. The essential fatty acids can't be made in the body, so they need to be supplied in our food. The key lies in the amount and proportion of these fats that we include in our diet.

A little bit of chemistry might explain why this is so important. Fats consist of different lengths of carbon atoms with hydrogen atoms attached. In the case of saturated fats, all of the carbon atoms have hydrogen atoms attached, there being no double bonds.

With monounsaturated fats, there is only one double-bond. Along with saturated fats, the mono-unsaturated fats are very stable and have higher boiling points when subject to heating.

The terms omega-3 and omega 6 fatty acids denote the carbon atom on which the first double-bond is found, as these essential fatty acids both have multiple double-bonds. The vast difference between them is the chemical pathways they follow.

Omega-3 causes an anti-inflammatory response, while omega-6 is pro-inflammatory. Knowing the significance of inflammation in chronic illness, and getting the balance right between these two essential fatty acids, is of utmost importance.

Added to this, the presence of double-bonds allows for more oxidative opportunities with the generation of free radicals which damages the cells. Excessive free radicals are known to be linked to chronic degenerative illnesses such as cardiovascular disease, autoimmune disease, and cancers.

The addition of antioxidants in the diet in foods such as goji berries, blueberries, pecans, and artichokes, to name a few, quench these free radicals and thereby stop the damage.

Saturated fats are foods such as butter, cream, ghee, and coconut oil. Because these fats are stable and not open to oxidation, they don't cause inflammation, which is one of the contributors to type 2 diabetes, obesity, and heart disease.

Slightly different, monounsaturated fats come in abundance in foods like olive oil, avocado, and certain nuts and seeds such as macadamia nuts, almonds, cashews, and pecans. Nut butters, such as cashew butter and almond butter, also join the mono group.

Foods containing omega-3 and omega-6 fatty acids contribute significantly to metabolic health on many levels. Both are essential in the diet because the body does not produce them, meaning they must be acquired in food. The secret is the balance between these two categories of fatty acids and how they affect our health.

Dietary items rich in omega-3 fatty acids include fish (especially cold-water species such as salmon, mackerel, and sardines), seaweeds, seeds such as chia and flax, and spices like oregano, cloves, and basil.

Foods high in omega-6 fatty acids include sunflower and safflower oil, grape-seed oil, and corn oil. The list of oils goes on, but many of them have been added to highly processed foods. These oils are essential in the correct balance, but are also pro-inflammatory and easily oxidized, thus requiring carefully controlled portions.

Tricky buggers, omega-6 fatty acids are essential to good health on the one hand, but inflammatory and antithetical to good health on the other. What's crucial is that they be consumed in balance with the anti-inflammatory omega-3 fatty acids.

Humans evolved consuming a diet with a 1:1 ratio of omega-6 to omega-3 fatty acids, yet today the average American diet runs a 15:1 ratio of inflammatory to anti-inflammatory, with a net effect that the body is being inundated with high levels of inflammation.

Health Watch recommends a reduction in the ratio to 4:1. It is estimated this reduction could reduce by 70% secondary cardiovascular mortality. Coupled with obesity, which further contributes to inflammation, the imbalance of omegas results in a deadly cocktail for cardiovascular disease. This imbalance is something **The *Fast* Diabetes Solution**™ resolves.

In connection with this subject, I was inspired to listen to the work of Dr. Aseem Malhotra, a British cardiologist, in the movie *The Big Fat Fix*. There he shares with us his passion for the Mediterranean diet and lifestyle, promoting a wide range of fresh vegetables, fish, olive oil, butter, and coconut oil, which he calls a "superfood."

The fine doctor addresses in particular what he describes as the three misconceptions of heart disease: (1) that dietary fat causes the narrowing of arteries, (2) that the narrowing or blockage of the arteries leads to heart attack, and (3) that reversal of the condition leading to heart attack takes a long time.

Instead, he assures us, it is inflammation that is at the core of heart disease — not dietary fat. Accordingly, he recommends four or more tablespoons of olive oil daily (of the cold-pressed extra virgin variety), such as adding olive oil to your salads or vegetables, frying eggs in olive oil and butter, and so on.

Collectively, these oils will pacify the inflammation present in the blood vessels. Thus, Dr. Malhotra tells us, by incorporating the Mediterranean-style diet — high portions of anti-inflammatory fats, low portions of carbs, moderate protein and lots of fresh salad and vegetables — heart disease can be reversed with the results evident in weeks.

I find this kind of information very exciting: dietary changes that can bring about reversal of both type 2 diabetes and heart disease at the same time over a short period following a yummy diet. With these huge myths debunked, let's do a few quick exercises before getting to the *Fast* **Diabetes Solution**.

Action

Have you been basing your diet on any of the food and dietary myths described in this chapter? If so, list them out.

Once you list them out, make a second list of foods that you think would be healthy substitutes for those you just eliminated.

Keep track of the results:

Chapter 4
THE PROBLEM

> "We cannot solve problems with the same
> thinking we used when we created them."
>
> — Albert Einstein

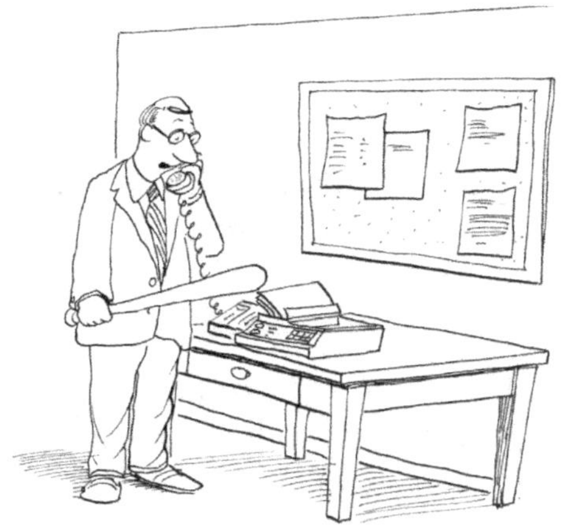

"Are you sure that hitting it
with a baseball bat will work?"

Information

Even with these myths debunked, you might be
asking: as an illness, how does type 2 diabetes work,
and what is the process that has enabled it to become
the world's fastest-growing disease? Put another
way, what is the problem? To answer these questions,
let's look more carefully at the exact process
involved.

The Process

First and foremost, type 2 diabetes is a dietary illness. As I have already discussed, it is driven by the hormone insulin, which is produced by the pancreas, with the subsequent development of insulin resistance. The pancreas is an organ located behind the stomach, and it plays a major role in your metabolism — that is, in the way your body turns digested food into energy.

When you eat, insulin is released from your pancreas. All foods cause some insulin response, but the response is highest with the ingestion of carbohydrates, or carbs; this is because carbs, in turn, break down into glucose and thus elevate glucose levels in the blood. The amount of insulin produced at any given time depends on the Glycemic Index (GI) of the carbs and the quantity of the carbohydrate you've ingested (the Glycemic Load).

Naturally, the volume of insulin released by the pancreas is greater with high-GI (high glycemic) carbohydrates. These carbs cause a rapid rise in blood glucose and therefore require higher levels of insulin to transport the glucose. By contrast, consuming normal portions of protein only causes a moderate rise in insulin and a small increase in blood glucose levels. (Note: the consumption of large amounts of protein does elicit an undesirable blood glucose response.)

By sharp contrast, any associated fat only elicits a small, insulin response, which is another plus for fat.

Depending on the composition of your meal, the pancreas will release a certain volume of insulin into the blood. Insulin and glucose then join hands and travel via the bloodstream to the billions of cells located throughout your body (we have about 37.2 trillion cells in all), where the cells utilize the glucose as energy.

The glucose is also stored in the liver in the form of glycogen to be used when energy is needed. Since your cells and liver can only store so much glucose, when the saturation point is reached the excess glucose remains in the blood. Insulin then pushes this excess glucose to the other form of energy: fat. It is through this process that you gain weight.

But you cannot think of weight only by what you see. That's because your weight resides, not only in your love handles or muffin tops visible in the mirror, but also internally in and around the abdomen, as visceral fat. As visceral fat, it fills your abdominal cavity and penetrates your surrounding organs, especially the liver. If you've heard of the diagnosis of a "fatty liver", now you know where it comes from.

While a fatty liver predisposes you to debilitating conditions such as cirrhosis and cancer of the liver, what is most pertinent here is that it's also a highly-accurate predictor of the development of type 2 diabetes. With more and more insulin resistance and more and more fat being stored in your fatty abdomen, eventually, your pancreas clogs up and interferes with your beta cells, whose job secreting insulin is hampered.

In a way of speaking, it is insulin resistance, therefore, that is making us fat. Think of insulin as a storage hormone pushing glucose into cells and, when that is no longer possible, creating fat for storage. When we eat excess carbs, i.e., junk food, fast food, and salty sugary sweets, we are constantly causing an insulin spike from our pancreas. Since our cells can no longer take in more glucose, their storage capacity being full they are resistant to the receipt of more glucose from the blood.

As a result, more insulin is released to cope with the excess blood glucose that the cells cannot absorb, resulting in more insulin resistance which in turn causes more insulin to be released. This in turn creates fat for which, unfortunately, the body provides unlimited storage. In the end, you can easily find yourself swirling in a vicious circle of insulin production, insulin resistance, and fat accumulation.

Welcome to obesity.

The Culprits

With this in mind, let's identify the culprits working behind the scenes to produce the primary villain: Insulin Resistance. Here they are:

1. Highly processed diets (including processed foods and processed sugar);

2. Excess carbohydrates (including fast food, most packaged snacks, candy bars, ice cream, sweets, puddings, potatoes, bread, pasta, and rice);

3. Eating too much too often at the wrong times, and;

4. Fructose (including HFCS contained in many processed foods).

Tell me something I didn't know, you might be thinking. But it bears emphasis since you're reading this book: all of these culprits — bar none — lead to increased insulin resistance, increased fat accumulation and storage, more fatty organs such as fatty liver and fatty pancreas, and, ultimately, beta cell dysfunction and type 2 diabetes, obesity, and heart disease.

Simple as that.

Sugar

We think of sugar as table sugar, the white and brown crystals that we add to our food and drinks for sweetness, without giving it a second thought. But it is much more than a harmless sweetener. Much more.

At the food factories, sugar is covertly added to almost all processed foods, from the obvious ones like children's cereal to the less obvious like bottled ketchup, salad dressings, and soups. The average American male adult consumes 21 added teaspoons of sugar every day (or about 336 calories). That's enough to fill a small drinking glass (try it). And for most people, one in five calories consumed comes from processed food.

Put more bluntly, table sugar and sugar added in the factory to processed food makes you fat, rots your teeth, and increases both inflammation and insulin resistance, thereby leading to pre-diabetes, type 2 diabetes, obesity and heart disease. Yet the "poison" we can't get enough of, lacks in any valuable nutrients of any kind and on its best day constitutes plain, empty calories.

So, what is sugar exactly and why is it such a problem?

Table or added sugar is a disaccharide, which technically is two sugars, glucose and fructose, joined together. Glucose is rapidly absorbed into the blood causing a rise in our blood sugar/glucose, which instantly causes an insulin response. This increased volume of blood glucose is then transported to cells throughout the body to be used as energy, stored for fuel in glycogen, or stored as excessive fat.

Enter fructose, the other portion of the sugar molecule. Fructose does not trigger an insulin response and unlike glucose has nowhere to go except to the liver, where the excess is stored as fat. How much fructose, you might ask, can a liver handle?

Not nearly as much as the average Western diet offers, that's for sure. Indeed, in his article "A New Paradigm of Insulin Resistance," Dr. Jason Fung reveals that fructose's contribution is far worse than the effect of glucose. To emphasize the point, he states that fructose's contribution to insulin resistance is 20 times that of glucose — due to the size and capacity of the liver to take in fructose compared to the trillions of cells in the body that deal with glucose. So, when HFCS is used by food-makers as the cheaper alternative to sugar, which historically has been the case, we have the formula for an epidemic.

Sadly, the economic forces that led to the use of HFCS as a cheaper, sweeter substitute for sugar in processed foods have done no one a service but subsidized U.S. corn growers. Instead, it has invisibly pushed our diet down a path to insulin resistance, obesity, type 2 diabetes, and heart disease at an unprecedented rate.

But please, do not confuse the fructose of processed sugar and HFCS with the fructose in natural fruit, vegetables, nuts, seeds, and legumes. Typically the fructose in fruit is not a dietary problem unless it is consumed in excessive amounts. The fructose in fruits and veggies combines with fiber and many nutrients to add value to our diet. It is the concentrated fructose found in HFCS and virtually all fruit drinks and soda pop that is the big problem. And there is very little fructose in nuts and seed.

Interestingly, as far back as 1972 British physiologist and nutritionist John Yudkin FRSC, the founding Professor of the Department of Nutrition at Queen Elizabeth College in London, exposed the harm caused by sugar to human dietary health. However, as so often happens, he was ridiculed by the industry whose vested interests were under attack (Big Food and Big Sugar, most notably), and then largely ignored by a medical profession blindly following conventional wisdom.

Undoubtedly, the controversy surrounding Professor Yudkin's findings resulted not only for his unpopular scientific findings, but also the fantastic title of his book, *Pure, White and Deadly*, which was released by Robert H. Lustig under the even more caustic title, *Pure, White and Deadly: How Sugar Is Killing Us and What We Can Do to Stop It.*

Type 2 Diabetes – The Mainstream Pills Approach

Now that I have fingered the culprits, let's examine how mainstream medicine addresses type 2 diabetes.

Almost daily I encounter a common scenario from my clients newly-diagnosed with diabetes or pre-diabetes: they are firmly advised to lose weight and exercise to reduce their blood glucose levels. Almost no dietary guidance is given, except some are told to see a dietician.

When following that advice, one of my clients reported that her dietician told her to snack on rice cakes. Surprised, I inquired whether the dietician had given her any GI advice. She looked at me blankly. Clearly her dietician had no idea that rice cakes were not suitable for a diabetic or anyone seeking to consume low-GI, highly-nutritional foods.

Neither was aware that rice cakes have a very high GI despite being light to the touch, eliciting a rapid insulin response. Moreover, to a diabetic, snacks should be discouraged. Curtailing insulin resistance requires longer periods of time between episodes of insulin production. If you eat high-GI foods, and keep pumping glucose into your bloodstream, your body produces more insulin to deal with it — the opposite of what you're trying to achieve.

Because physicians typically leave their patients to their own pre-existing bad dietary habits, what often happens is that several weeks or months later the patients return to their physicians (whether thinner or not) with sky-high blood glucose levels that are off the charts — often worse than when they first tested.

At that time, physicians will normally put their patients on a pharmaceutical medication such as Metformin. Metformin lowers your liver glucose production, increases uptake of glucose into your muscle cells and delays the absorption of glucose from the intestines after eating but unless your insulin resistance is also being addressed, higher levels of Metformin will be required, often accompanied by nausea and diarrhea.

The advantage of Metformin is that it doesn't increase insulin levels. However, when Metformin starts to falter and usually it will, a sulfonylurea drug such as Diabeta or Amaryl will be added to the mix, putting you on two meds. This new drug will stimulate your pancreas to produce even more insulin with even more potential adverse side-effects.

With two meds at work, the extra insulin your body produces now moves your excess blood glucose into excess fat storage. And this is the inevitable cycle: each additional drug gives good results for a while, but as your diabetes progresses, more drugs with different actions will typically be added. When the maelstrom of meds runs its course, as it often does, many of you will find yourselves put on insulin injections — all while you continue to pile on the weight. How depressing!

Not to mention, the expense of treatment and the side-effects involved continue to mount, leaving your insulin resistance raging unabated. That's because your treatment is aimed at your blood glucose levels, while beneath it all the true culprits — insulin resistance and visceral fat — are not being addressed at all, and your eyes, kidneys, heart, and blood vessels are all paying a massive price.

That price is not only in bad health, but in dollars at the pharmacy counter and potential bodily disability such as blindness and limb amputation. Therefore, in my opinion, much of the massive amount of money being directed to finance drug research would be much better spent educating everyone — physician, patients, policymakers, and the general public alike — on the essentials of a healthy diet, exercise, and stress management. This might help undo decades of incorrect dietary advice that has contributed mightily to this pandemic in the first place.

Unless and until we address these underlying causes, we cannot prevent, cure and reverse diabetes. Which is a serious challenge for conventional medicine and contemporary culture. Indeed, current medical guides addressing the type 2 diabetes typically describe it as a progressive disease requiring sustained long-term drug interventions, which as we now know does not address or lower insulin resistance.

In short, we need to stop treating this epidemic of dietary illness with a drug-based mindset and regime, limiting drugs to essential need only, and instead adopt a healthier diet and lifestyle.

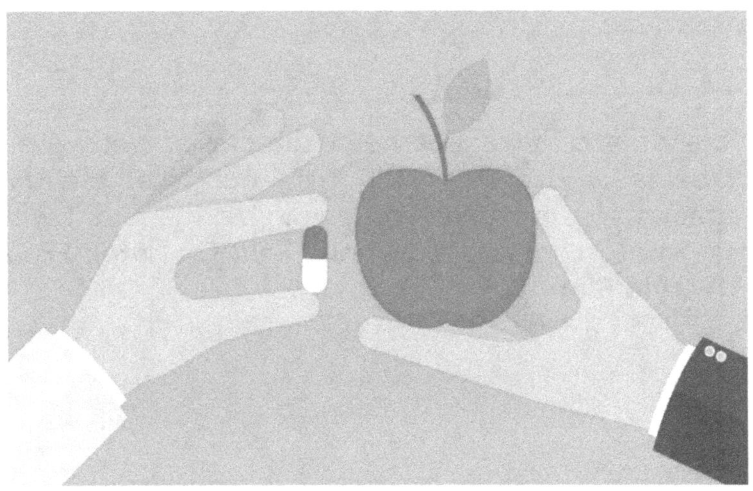

Action

When you were first diagnosed with pre-diabetes and/or type 2 diabetes, did your physician give you any directions on diet, e.g., eat less, avoid sugar, no carbs, reduce calories? If so, please indicate the advice in detail below:

Based on this advice, or left to your own to figure it out, what did you do, i.e., what old dietary habits did you stop and what new ones (if any) did you begin? Be specific.

Note: If you have not been diagnosed with pre-diabetes or diabetes, still write out what dietary regimen you have been following. At the end, I will ask you to compare it to your *Fast* **Diabetes-Free Lifestyle Plan**.

Chapter 5
THE RESEARCH

> "1,500 years ago, everybody knew the earth was
> the center of the universe. 500 years ago,
> everybody knew the earth was flat. And 15
> minutes ago, you knew that people were alone
> on this planet. Imagine what you'll know
> tomorrow."
>
> — *Men in Black*

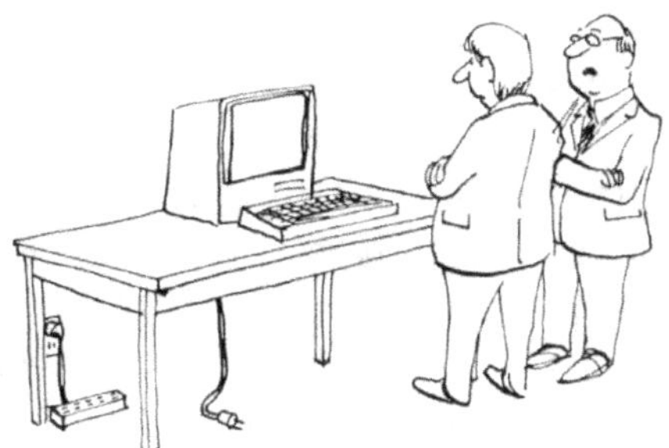

"It could be an expensive repair,
or it could just be the plug is out."

Information

This chapter collects some of the compelling research on diet, exercise, stress management, and type 2 diabetes that sparks our optimism and distills confidence in us that you can reverse your diabetes *Fast*, allowing you to embrace a new, healthier lifestyle and happier self.

Suzanne Ridley

The Research of Professor Roy Taylor – Reversing Your Diabetes

The ground-breaking diabetes research of Professor Roy Taylor of Newcastle University provides the foundation for our confidence that you can reverse your diabetes *Fast.* Here's the amazing story of how he discovered the road to type 2 diabetes reversal.

Over the years, Professor Taylor observed that bariatric surgery patients would afterward present marked improvements in their blood-sugar profiles. These are the patients who have an adjustable band placed around their stomach tops, literally shrinking their stomach capacity and severely reducing the amount of food they can consume.

According to the Professor, he expected that the morbidly-obese patients would undergo significant weight loss. What he did not expect was the significant drop in blood-sugar readings because, by definition, the surgery was a radical, non-dietary intervention. Armed with this knowledge, Professor Taylor conceived a specialized low-calorie diet of 800 calories per day for eight consecutive weeks, to test his hypothesis that weight reduction was the cause.

After scrupulously following the "8-week, low-cal diet" created by the Professor, volunteers reported substantial reductions of fat in their livers and pancreases. This reduction in fat enabled their bodies to restore healthy levels of insulin production that put their type 2 diabetes into remission. Three months later, some volunteers had put weight back on, but most maintained normal blood glucose levels.

As Professor Taylor gathered data from his clinical trials, he naturally wanted to classify the results. He did so by creating two simple designations: "Responders" and "Non-Responders." Each participant fell into one classification or the other, depending on how well he or she responded to this radical 800-calorie (low-calorie) diet.

Participants were deemed "Responders" if they succeeded in reversing their diabetic symptoms and reinstating their normal blood glucose levels and insulin production — in other words, if they cured or reversed their diabetes. Participants were deemed "Non-responders" if their symptoms were not fully reversed and returned to normal, i.e., if they continued to record above-normal blood glucose readings which still classified them as being diabetic, albeit improved.

Using this classification system, Professor Taylor found that the people most likely to be classified as "Responders" with total reversals had been diagnosed with type 2 diabetes for less than five years. But even for the "Non-responders" who remained diabetic, their blood glucose levels decreased, often significantly, an important benefit in and of itself.

But that's not all. For both groups, whether classified as "Responder" or "Non-responder," the risk of cardiovascular disease was greatly reduced. This is significant because cardiovascular disease is the leading cause of death for diabetics, with those aged 65 or older having a 68% chance of dying from cardiovascular disease. Thus, by significantly decreasing the risk of cardiovascular disease for all participants, the new diet delivered a prolonged and healthier life for all who followed it.

Which is not to say that "Responders" only consisted of diabetics of five years or less. Some participants with 10+ years as diabetics also completely reversed their diabetes, joyously joining the ranks of the "Responders." Though length of time with diabetes was a leading factor, it turned out not to be the sole determinant. Theoretically, therefore, any person with diabetes could become a "Responder" and all diabetics enjoyed enormous improvements in health that will make them healthier, happier and live longer, all other factors equal.

Spurred by these findings, in 2013, Diabetes UK, a non-profit enterprise devoted to battling diabetes, awarded their largest-ever research grant (£2.4 million) to Professor Taylor and his colleague Professor Mike Lean of the University of Glasgow. The award tasked them with comparing the relative long-term impact on type 2 diabetics of Taylor's low-calorie diet, with the best diabetic care currently being offered.

The goal of DiRECT (the common name given to the ensuing Diabetes Remission Clinical Trial) was to determine if the intensive 8-week diet plan followed by an intensive weight management regimen could stop, reverse and cure type 2 diabetes. Since final results of the trial will not be available until next October 2018, Diabetes UK is withholding formal endorsement until that time. The writing, however, is on the wall, given the significant prior clinical results and the growing consensus among physicians and nutrition experts that reduced weight can reverse diabetes.

I am highly indebted to Professor Taylor for essentially discovering that the world of diabetes is not flat — i.e., that type 2 diabetes can be reversed, cured, and eradicated through an 8-week low-calorie diet. His findings represent a paradigm shift in the way that diabetes and diabetes prognosis should be viewed, adding to the burgeoning weight of evidence, no pun intended, that simply losing weight — fat clogging your vital organs — can reverse type 2 diabetes for many people. It need no longer be *until death do us part.*

There is also a greater truth in these findings as well. Not only did weight reduction produce these results, the 8-week crash diet led to reduced insulin resistance (or, to put it another way, improved insulin management). With food consumption drastically reduced, the body had longer periods of time in which production and use of insulin was not at play.

As research continues into what actually causes insulin resistance, we must shift our focus from caloric restriction to reduction of carbohydrates, especially processed sugar, HFCS, and fructose. Armed with this knowledge, all type 2 diabetics have at their fingertips the potential to reverse their diabetes or pre-diabetic conditions...and indeed, this is happening every day.

When combined with my own 40+ years of experience as a pharmacist working in the trenches daily, this new paradigm truly opened my heart, as there is now hope and optimism for the tens of millions of people worldwide whose conditions can be cured or substantially improved. That hope lies at the core of this book. And with that hope in mind, let's take a look at some additional, related research findings that further bolster our optimism.

The Glycemic Index (GI) Research of Dr. David Jenkins

In 1981, Dr. David Jenkins and his colleagues introduced the concept of the Glycemic Index ("GI") that I referenced earlier in the book. As you'll recall, GI shows the rate at which different carbohydrates break down into glucose and influence blood glucose levels. Foods with a high GI value increase blood glucose levels rapidly, causing an insulin spike, while those with a lower GI value affect blood glucose more slowly.

This phenomenon — the differing results of high and low GI — was totally at odds with the prevailing view at the time: that all carbohydrates were created equal, and that a diet based on equal carbohydrate exchange — one portion of potatoes for one portion of fruit — is what the doctor ordered. Instead, Dr. Jenkins' research showed that potatoes and bread had a much higher GI than their brothers and sisters in the sugary snacks aisles, such as fruits and chocolate bars. Until then, sugar had been seen as the primary high-GI culprit.

Time and more research prevailed with countries throughout the world recommending the low-GI approach to gain improved blood glucose control. We now have over 2,000 foods tested for their GI value due to the work of such committed professionals such as Professor Jennie Brand-Miller — of Sydney University's Science Department. Thus, while sugar is not our friend — and often is our enemy — we do need to adjust the needle ever so slightly so that it hovers squarely atop the vast category of all high-GI foods — whether natural, processed, additives, sweet from sugar, or otherwise.

A small word of caution. Just because a food is low-GI does not mean it can be consumed without rational limit. The volume of food you consume indisputably plays an important role in your diet and insulin management as well. If you now think you can load up with a plate full of pasta, think again. The volume of carbohydrate involved (the Glycemic Load) will also cause a high insulin response. This is so despite pasta having a low to medium GI.

Put another way, the truth about carbohydrates is that they are NOT an essential part of our diet (as suggested by them being placed at the base of the Food Pyramid). Though many of us enjoy eating them (often spurred by bad habits established earlier in life), we can in truth live happily by taking a smart approach: keeping our carb load low and using the glycemic index to guide our choice of carbs when we do choose — carefully and selectively — to eat them. (For example, choosing basmati rice over jasmine rice, knowing the former will have a vastly more favorable effect on our blood glucose level.)

It would be wonderful to be able to follow the GI and select carbs wisely... and all would be well. Unfortunately, life is rarely that simple. As I have discussed, processed sugar and fructose play a major role in the development of insulin resistance and, therefore, type 2 diabetes. This is despite sugar having a medium GI rating and fructose landing in the low range. The GI is a great tool, but it needs to be used wisely.

The Research on Inflammation

For over a decade, scientists have been looking at the role of inflammation in causing insulin resistance. Although not all questions have been answered, it has become clear that obese individuals often present with chronic, low-grade inflammation.

The explanation is straightforward. Insulin binds to receptor sites on the surface of your body's muscles, organs, nerves and other cells. These cells respond by taking up glucose, thus removing that glucose from your blood and transforming it into energy. However, when inflammation is present in your adipose or fat cells, chemicals such as cytokines are produced, acting as mediators. Because cytokines are inflammatory they adversely affect the signaling of insulin, disabling the ability of your cells to respond. This, in turn, contributes to insulin resistance.

As obesity climbs, so do the number of people afflicted with chronic illnesses that result from obesity and the consequent inflammation. Adopting a nutritious, balanced diet, eating smaller portions, and eating less often are the best places to start.

Good medicine — and common sense — suggest your diet should include healthy portions of foods which reduce inflammation. These are foods high in omega-3 fatty acids, such as fish, nuts and seeds; good oils like olive and macadamia oil; butter and coconut oil; green leafy vegetables; and fruits such as blueberries and strawberries.

Indeed, because of the ill effects it causes, inflammation has become the new buzz word in medicine. Inflammation and insulin resistance lie at the basis of chronic health conditions. We all know about the swollen, inflamed joints of arthritis because we can see puffy feet and limbs with our own two eyes. But the more dangerous process going on deep inside our body is the one we cannot see — one of chronic, low-grade inflammation occurring around our major organs and even in our blood vessels.

Inflammation presents an even bigger worry because it is the condition that contributes to diabetes, cardiovascular disease, fatty liver disease, inflammatory airways disease, and dementia, only to name a few. Where does this inflammation come from, you may ask? I have already identified the role of obesity, but for more answers let's turn to the contributory role of gut health.

The Research on Gut Health

Of growing importance to all aspects of health is your gut. We all know when we are constipated or bloated because we experience discomfort, which typically passes either momentarily or over the next 12 to 24 hours. But what's housed there — what shouldn't be and what should be — these are the vital considerations that we will explore next.

The gut is home to trillions of diverse bacteria, most of them residing in the gastrointestinal tract. As such, they impact your health in many ways. Since healthy gut microbes increase the number of white blood cells that fight disease, one specific impact is on your immune system. Unhealthy levels of gut microbes are associated with all sorts of unhealthy conditions, including obesity, eczema, asthma, allergies, autoimmune disorders, and even mood disorders.

I am confident that having a healthy gut is central to general health and well-being, and as knowledge of the gut microbiome increases, the importance of this composition will also increase.

Given this state of affairs, it comes as no surprise that gut health might play a substantial role in contracting, managing and reversing type 2 diabetes. This belief led a group of Russian scientists, including Dr. Elena Kostryukova and Maria Vakhitova, to investigate the gut bacteria levels and varieties residing in victims of pre-diabetes and diabetes. Their findings, published in *Endocrinology Connections*, established a demonstrable link between glucose intolerance and three different bacteria: Blautia, Serratia, and Akkermansia.

In short, their investigation demonstrated that people with diabetes or pre-diabetes report significantly higher levels of all three gut bacteria. Therefore, the assumption is that these bacteria are causing an immune response in their hosts. Presumably, the intestinal bacteria is creating toxins which in turn provoke inflammation in the gut which in turn affects the body's metabolism, increasing insulin resistance. Clearly, we need to pay particular attention to improving gut health and managing gut microbiota (the composition of bacteria living in the intestines) as part of our journey to reversing diabetes and achieving a lifetime of better health.

There is no doubt the food you eat has a powerful influence over your gut microbiota. Eating fresh fruit and vegetables, chia seeds, flaxseeds, beans, and grains — especially foods high in fiber — are all valuable sources of soluble fiber, which serves as food source for healthy, beneficial bacteria. These foods are described as prebiotic. Fermented foods — such as sauerkraut, kimchi, pickles, kefir, homemade yogurt, and kombucha — all provide probiotics, thus helping maintain healthy gut colonies.

One way to obtain a healthy gut is to add bitterness to your diet, as it stimulates your digestion. Unfortunately, the standard western diet is sadly lacking in bitter foods like bitter melon, rocket, dandelion, endives, and watercress. All stimulate digestive juices, starting with salivation, allowing food to be chewed and digested more easily. This commences the process of digestion, increasing the flow of stomach acid and enzymes which break down food for better absorption and increase bile flow in the liver and gallbladder. As a result, by the time the food reaches the intestines, digestion is well underway.

Diets and lifestyles heaped in processed food, processed sugar, HFCS, table salt, chemical preservatives, alcohol, stress, and antibiotic use — all negatively impact gut health and foster overpopulation of unfriendly bacteria. Changing your old diet and lifestyle and replacing them with a healthy, holistic life-affirming one will give you a happier gut in the process. And a happier gut will equate to a happier you.

The Research on Obesity

The Obesity Society knows obesity. According to their website, "Obesity is one of the most pervasive, chronic diseases in need of new strategies for medical treatment and prevention. As a leading cause of United States mortality, morbidity, disability, healthcare utilization and healthcare costs, the high prevalence of obesity continues to strain the United States healthcare system."

Obesity, of course, starts with food — how much you eat, how little, and what. But of equal importance is *when*. And though we often eat unthinkingly, a bad habit acquired by western society over the last century, the science and biology of eating — of food intake — is actually quite complex, requiring careful thought and examination.

Believe it or not, food operates on a much higher level than tasting good or bad. Its smell, taste, texture, and temperature all trigger cognitive and emotional responses within us, as well as providing our brains with metabolic and autonomic information. Some food tells you to eat more when you shouldn't, while other food tells you to eat little or nothing when you should eat loads. For example, fast foods, candy, and white bread all tell you to eat more, when you should eat less.

When something so important as diet, food intake and obesity get out of hand, due largely to culturally-instilled bad dietary habits, it is not surprising that entire populations of people are adversely affected. Just ask the tens of millions of Americans with diabetes or pre-diabetes or the millions who are obese.

And obesity comes at a big cost. Not only to the individual, but to society. The U.S. Center for Disease Control estimates over 112,000 U.S. deaths per year result from obesity, with the "obese-challenged" at risk for 30+ chronic health conditions, including: type 2 diabetes, high cholesterol, hypertension, gallstones, heart disease, fatty liver disease, sleep apnea, GORD, stress incontinence, heart failure, degenerative joint disease, birth defects, miscarriages, respiratory conditions, and cancers.

Not surprisingly, healthcare costs to America revolving around obesity are fast approaching $200 billion annually. This doesn't include the mistreatment, prejudice, and abuse of the obese that runs contrary to our twig-thin, curved-figure model-worshipping culture. But obesity is by no means unique to America, spreading its largess worldwide just like type 2 diabetes.

High Body Mass Index (BMI) — that function of height and weight — now ranks among the world's greatest health concerns, joining the axis of malnutrition (ironically), high cholesterol, unsafe sex, iron deficiency, smoking, alcohol abuse, drug abuse, and unsafe water in total global burden of disease and disaster.

On a biological level, obesity is simply excess adipose — or fatty — tissue amassing itself within the human body. Whether the volume of fatty tissue in your system has crossed the line into obesity, becoming excess, is determined by several measurements. The most common is the BMI (body mass index).

Obesity, therefore, lies in the target of any program to reverse, cure, and live a diabetes-free life and lifestyle. Make no mistake, obesity is a hormonal disease governed by insulin resistance and hormones that regulate appetite. So let's explore further the important role in dietary health played by "hunger hormones."

The Research on the Hunger Hormones

There are three major "hunger hormones": Ghrelin, Leptin, and Neuropeptide Y (NPY).

When Ghrelin is secreted in the stomach, it stimulates our appetite. Levels are high before a meal and drop after a meal. Ghrelin levels are surprisingly low in the morning even though we may not have eaten for 12 to 14 hours and are highest at night. Hence, our desire for a midnight snack.

Leptin is produced by fat cells, and is the satiety hormone tasked with sending messages to the brain to stop eating when we've had enough to eat. This hormone has been found to be inhibited in the obese, which means they are receiving a weaker signal to stop eating. This is termed leptin resistance.

NPY is a hormone mainly found in the brain. It has a potent stimulating effect on appetite, especially when carbohydrates are present, and it delays feelings of fullness. It is mainly released when calories are restricted and levels of leptin are low.

So why do calorie-restricted diets ultimately result in a yo-yo effect? Here's why. Dr. Jason Fung explains that when calories are reduced there is a corresponding decrease in the metabolic rate. Reductions of calories by 30% will quickly elicit a decrease in metabolic rate of 30%. The body is conserving energy to carry out the necessary bodily functions relating to breathing, heartbeat, kidney function, heat production. Ghrelin levels are increased, making us feel hungry; leptin levels drop, so the message to our brain of fullness is lessened; and if that wasn't enough, the low leptin levels cause NPY to kick in, thus stimulating feelings of hunger.

On top of that, hormones are stubborn. It can take as long as a year after any substantial weight loss for your hormones to get the message and change their engrained response cycles. When you look closely at the hormone dynamics, you see why it isn't only about having the willpower to diet or reduce calories. Your own hormones are working against you and your weight loss.

But hang on a minute, let's be clear about one thing in the event your mind is oversimplifying things. Though caloric restriction triggers your hunger hormones, remember that calories *per se* are not the reason we accumulate fat. The reason you accumulate fat is the other hormone: insulin. Keep your eye on the doughnut, not the hole, as they say, no pun intended, because by doing this you realize the true villain is carbohydrates, which more than anything else increases your insulin levels and leads to dangerous accumulation of fat.

All of this very fairly gives us a message: don't be so hard on yourself — be empowered with the knowledge of smart food choices and that your hard work will pay off, eventually making your new lifestyle in health easier and easier.

Which leads us back to your hunger hormones, which are triggered by much more than diet, i.e., food or the lack of it. All three hunger hormones are also influenced dramatically by sleep deprivation and stress, which we will discuss later.

But with the role of calories still swirling in our minds, let's turn to fasting.

The Research of Intermittent Fasting and Time-Restricted Feeding

Fasting dates back to the beginning of living things. In the course of existence, nature preternaturally triggers fasting in times of illness or stress. Whether human or animal, the DNA in living organisms is hard-wired to find rest, balance, and energy-conservation during critical times.

The use of fasting as a healing method found praise from early thinkers like Hippocrates, Plato, Socrates, and Aristotle. One of the fathers of western medicine, Paracelsus, said: "Fasting is the greatest remedy — the remedy within."

Religious and spiritual groups have also long embraced fasting, particularly during the equinoxes, spring and fall, and every major religion has engaged it for spiritual purposes — from Christianity and Judaism to Islam, Buddhism, Hinduism, and the Yogis.

In the late 1800s, Dr. Herbert Shelton reported on the fasts of over 40,000 people. This led him to conclude that "fasting must be recognized as a fundamental and radical process that is older than any other mode of caring for the sick organism, for it is employed on the plane of instinct."

A study at the USC Leonard Davis School of Gerontology found 71 out of 100 people on a "fasting mimicking" regime substantially improved their cardiovascular risk factors (blood pressure, inflammation, etc.) while reducing both fat and levels of IGF-1, a hormone that affects metabolism.

Another human study published in Lifestyle Management to Reduce Diabetes/Cardiovascular risk demonstrated the huge benefits of intermittent fasting for type 2 diabetics. They found fasting reduced blood sugar by 3–6%, while fasting insulin was reduced by a whopping 20–31%.

When depriving the body of food (even for small periods of time), lower blood glucose and insulin levels ensue which then allow a rebalancing of the body's capacity to utilize stored energy and normalize your insulin response. ***This single process is the master key to unlocking the shackles to insulin resistance, visceral fat, and curing type 2 diabetes.***

The 2015 study "Effect of intermittent fasting and refeeding on insulin action in healthy men" published in the *Journal of Applied Physiology* also revealed even in non-diabetic men that intermittent fasting increases the rate of glucose uptake. Translated in general terms, this means intermittent fasting reduces insulin resistance and improves insulin sensitivity, even if the subject is relatively healthy and does not have high levels of insulin resistance to begin with.

More evidence to support how effective intermittent fasting can work effectively as a natural weapon against diabetes comes from Professor Valter Longo of biological sciences at the USC Dornsife College of Letters, Arts and Sciences, who discovered in a study on mice that intermittent fasting resulted in the regeneration of pancreatic cells in both type 1 and type 2 diabetic mice.

According to Longo, "Cycles of a fasting-mimicking diet and a normal diet essentially reprogrammed non-insulin-producing cells into insulin-producing cells," which I might add is extraordinary for its implications for long-term diabetics.

Professor Longo further observed: "By activating the regeneration of pancreatic cells, we were able to rescue mice from late-stage type 1 and type 2 diabetes. We also reactivated insulin production in human pancreatic cells from type 1 diabetes patients."

Wow!

This means that the common deterioration of beta cell function to produce insulin in the later stages of type 2 diabetes shows the potential of being fully reversed through an intermittent fasting model of treatment. This groundbreaking discovery offers those type 2 diabetics who find themselves in the later and more perilous stages of type 2 diabetes — the ones less likely to fully benefit by Dr. Taylor's

800-calories fasting regime — enormous optimism for their own diabetic recovery.

Of course, like every other radical health departure, common sense dictates that you first seek your doctor's input if you have any existing health issues or any questions about adopting a radically-new fasting or dietary practice. Better safe than sorry.

In sum, there is no question that fantastic results have been and can be achieved through a program of fasting. However, for diabetics on insulin or medication which can cause hypoglycemia, ***this should never be attempted without the careful involvement of your physician*** because your medication will need to be adjusted as your blood glucose levels drop.

The Research of Dr. Panda

If forgoing food for long periods of time is just out of the question for you, then you may be fascinated by Dr. Satchidananda Panda's research of Time-Restricted Feeding. Dr. Panda, a Professor of Biology at the Regulatory Biology Laboratory of the Panda Institute, highlights the importance not only of what we eat, but *when* we eat it.

Most of you have heard about the circadian clock or master clock which governs your biorhythms and manages your sleep-wake cycle. At the core of the circadian clock are daylight and darkness — in a word, light. Not only does light influence your sleep patterns, it also ticks in your liver, triggering organ function similarly to the presence or absence of food or drink.

Not surprisingly, what he observed about the liver is that it works most effectively and efficiently when the internal liver clock starts ticking. Because that also is the time the body is most insulin-sensitive, that's when the liver works best to break down fats and aid in the digestion process.

As time passes, the effectiveness of the process diminishes. Based on studies with mice, Dr. Panda hypothecates that the liver starts running out of steam as the day progresses, thus suggesting a 12-hour window within which all daily food consumption would ideally — and most proficiently — take place. Thus, if you take your first cup of coffee at 7 am, it might be best to stop eating at about 7 pm, or even squeeze the time further, starting at 8 am and ending at 6 pm. In other words, here's even more reason to banish the fatuous thought of the healthy midnight snack.

Conclusion

It may well feel like all this research is tedious, but the beauty of research is that it both deconstructs and simplifies, often sending us on an adventure of learning that lasts us a lifetime. In other words, if you're questioning anything I'm saying, dig in and research it yourself. Knowledge is dynamic. But, I am absolutely certain of one thing: if you follow the guiding solutions espoused in this book, complemented and adjusted by your own research if you so desire, you will come away healthier and happier.

Action

Summarize here the research you were aware of before reading this book (I have given you extra space):

Compare and contrast what you knew about research into insulin, fasting and such before reading this book, and what you have learned so far (again, I have given you extra space).

PART II: THE SOLUTION

Chapter 6
FASTING – THE *FAST* WAY TO RECOVERY

"Everyone has a doctor in him; we just have to help him in his work. The natural healing force within each one of us is the greatest force in getting well. To eat when you are sick, is to feed your sickness."

– Hippocrates

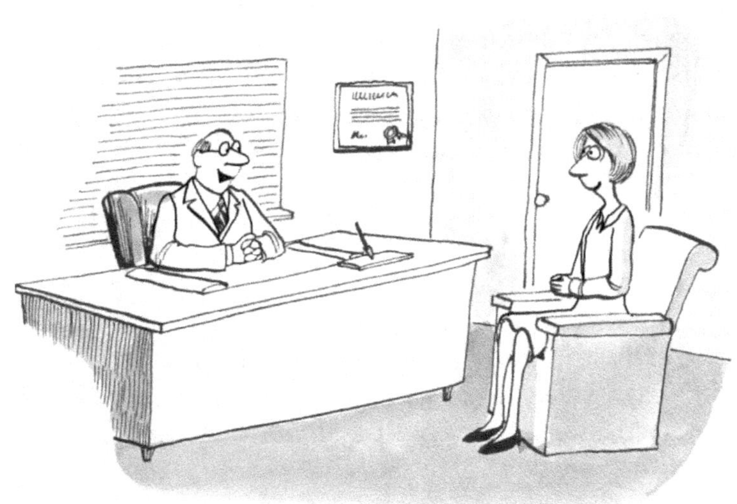

Information

Definitions of *Fast*. There are several. Here are two.

Fast 1: acting or moving or capable of acting or moving quickly.

Fast 2: to abstain from eating all or certain foods.

The first holistic principle of **The *Fast* Diabetes Solution** to stopping, reversing and curing your type 2 diabetes (or pre-diabetic symptoms) derives from the name of the book: fasting, which incorporates a bit of both definitions.

What does fasting involve?

The short answer is: abstinence from eating food while keeping well-hydrated. Allowable hydration are water, tea, coffee, or broths (bone or vegetable), with a dash of milk if desired but no sweetening agents of any kind. Extra salt should be added when fasting for longer periods of time, in the form of sea salt or Himalayan salt added to your water or broth.

As all food consumption causes some insulin response, consuming no food means no glucose is entering the blood and no insulin response is required, which is what takes place during fasting. For energy, the body naturally turns first to its excess glucose storage, and when the glucose stores are exhausted (after a couple of days) fat stores will be used to generate energy.

More specifically, the body extracts fat first from the liver and then the pancreas whose cells are freed up to go about their normal job unimpeded. With this process working for you, improvement in your diabetic symptoms will occur rapidly, also leading to the added bonus of a svelte new you.

What degree of fasting are we talking about? Intensely at first, and then intermittently over time. Or you might prefer to ease into the longer fasting periods by dipping your toes in first to test the waters.

How long must my fasting last?

There are several options to choose from. The option you choose depends on your mind-body makeup. Some people can do the super-*Fast* option, which is fasting for a week or more and feeling totally invigorated, finding it far easier than expected. If you choose this option, you will be strolling down the fastest known path to reversing your type 2 diabetes and eliminating pre-diabetic symptoms.

It surprises many people to find that the hunger they were so worried about dissipates drastically after day two. It will come and go in waves, but far less intensity. This correlates with the decrease in ghrelin (the hunger hormone) that is observed over three days of fasting.

However, not everyone will feel compelled to undertake the super-*Fast* approach the first time despite the profound and dramatic results. For you, one alternative is to pick two or three days each week instead — Monday, Wednesday, Friday; Tuesday Thursday; or maybe Sunday and Monday. Whatever combination works for your life schedule.

If that seems too much to tackle, the easiest approach is to find one day a week that you can dedicate to fasting continually for 24 continuous hours. Over this one day you will avoid all foods between dinner times — say, from dinner Monday night to dinner Tuesday night (24 hours). This day can change from week to week to fit your schedule.

If a full 24-hour day of fasting is still too daunting, then ratchet it back even further to a 16-hour fasting period lasting, for example, from 8 pm Saturday night through noon Sunday. Many of you may come close to doing that already. And if you think about it, all you're doing is shunning late-night snacks and having a late brunch. Very accessible and very doable, even for the faint of heart.

You can also be creative, mixing everything up as and when it suits you, your willpower, your food hormones, and your schedule. By this I mean, fast 24 hours one day a week for week one, 16 hours a day for one day a week during week two, two days here, three days there — whatever works!

Now, you might be asking, that's it? After reading all this way you're simply telling me to stop eating? Yes, in a way, that's it. Stop eating for the times involved. But like so many things in life, easier said than done, and of course there's more to it than that, as the fasting must be followed by a lifetime commitment to proper diet, exercise, and stress management.

But before we get to that, let's drill down on the specifics of how you'll go about your new fasting routine.

Routine for Intermittent Fasting

Having a routine makes the job easier. So let's break it down. With intermittent fasting, there are two types of days: those days and/or hours you are fasting, i.e., not eating and only hydrating, and those days and/or hours you are eating between fasting.

Let's take the non-fasting days and/or hours first. On the days you're not fasting, i.e., on the days or during the times you're eating, you'll need to follow these guidelines as rigorously as your mind and body will allow:

1. Eat a low-carb diet that keeps the demands on your insulin production low and your liver working to shed your fat (not burn newly-arriving carb calories, which is always its priority if you give it the chance).

2. Keep your focus on eating good quality protein, healthy fats, and lots of fresh vegetables and salad (we will give you a nice list of these later in the book).

3. Only eat during a limited, prescribed timeframe, preferably during a maximum 12-hour block, say between 7:00 pm and 7:00 am. The key is to reduce your insulin requirement daily for 12 continuous hours.

4. Needless to say, though I'll say it to reinforce it: NO SNACKING, NO PROCESSED FOODS, NO SUGAR, NO HIGH-GI CARBS, NO HIGH-FRUCTOSE FRUITS and NO HFCS

Four simple and basic steps, right? And the only difference between the super-**Fast** diet solution and the slower but still relatively fast alternatives is how quickly you will shed the pounds, evaporate inner fat, control inflammation and manage your metabolism.

No matter which **Fasting** routine you choose, you will undergo a visible and major lifestyle change in a relatively short period of time. And since all time is relative, compared to the slow deterioration of chronic pre-diabetes symptoms and type 2 diabetes, no matter what approach you take it will be **Fast** in every sense of the word.

We've come a long way, but some of you may now be asking, why not simply follow a low-calorie diet?

No, it is more complicated than that. This is where easier-said-than-done kicks in. The challenge lies in maintaining the weight loss after your intense fasting is complete.

Here's how it will unfold when you are calorie counting. At first, you will drop a load of weight and feel pretty good about yourself. You'll be lighter on your feet, you'll look thin in the mirror, your curves will start returning, your waist will shrink, and your old clothes will no longer fit. That's what all calorie-restricted diets do.

However, calorie-restricted diets per se do not focus on your insulin or insulin resistance. In many of these diets, carbs are allowed — which means you are still producing glucose from the daily consumption of carbs and thus still require insulin to be released from the pancreas to burn the glucose, rather than burn your fat.

With this type of dieting — dieting that focuses only on calories and not on insulin, insulin resistance, and carbohydrate consumption — your metabolic rate drops as your body conserves energy to carry out its functions. In other words, your body is still burning sugar for energy and secreting all the same hunger hormones in the same counter-productive way.

So, with this low-cal only form of dieting, if you are doing a workout at the gym, you will now have to double your efforts to get the same result because your body will not burn fat. In fact, even though you've altered your metabolic rate by consuming fewer calories, your body will decipher this, accustom itself to a low-calorie metabolic rate, and over time (despite eating fewer calories), your weight will return because your fat will return.

When someone exclaims they don't understand why the weight is piling back on, now: a) you know they are more than likely telling you the truth, and b) you know why: they are reducing their calories but not controlling their insulin and insulin resistance.

Now let's bring it back to fasting. When you fast, insulin levels are reduced there is no glucose being supplied for fuel and your body automatically and naturally turns to its fat storage for energy, burning fat rather than sugar. And there is no reduction in metabolic rate; quite the opposite: your resting metabolic rate increases as does your adrenalin, so you have more energy than ever before.

The Obesity Code

To stay on track, let's take a brief diversion back into the science. In his book *The Obesity Code*, Dr. Jason

Fung places insulin at the core of both type 2 diabetes and obesity. He argues persuasively that if we lower our exposure to insulin, reduced insulin resistance will follow.

Weight loss will be sustained, with insulin management being the key to resetting your metabolic clock. Reducing calories is a general approach, but reducing your consumption of carbohydrates is the core goal as this also eliminates the high insulin response that always follows carb intake.

Let's put it another way. Not all calories are created equally. Calories from eating protein and fat cause only a minimal insulin response, but calories consumed carbs do the opposite. Only reducing calories leaves insulin and insulin resistance unaddressed, such that insulin levels remain high despite fewer calories being consumed.

That is why **The *Fast* Diabetes Solution** takes a multi-prong approach that kicks off with fasting to get you a fast initial solution, but then turns to the critical holistic need to address diet, low-carb intake, exercise and stress control, all of which are still to come.

Action

Have you ever fasted before? If so, write down how and when you fasted.

What were the results of your fasting experience?

If you have never fasted, why not?

Now that you've read this chapter on fasting, what fasting routine do you think will be best for you, given your lifestyle and schedule?

Chapter 7
YOUR FASTING OPTIONS

"He who eats until he is sick must fast until he is well."

– Old English Proverb

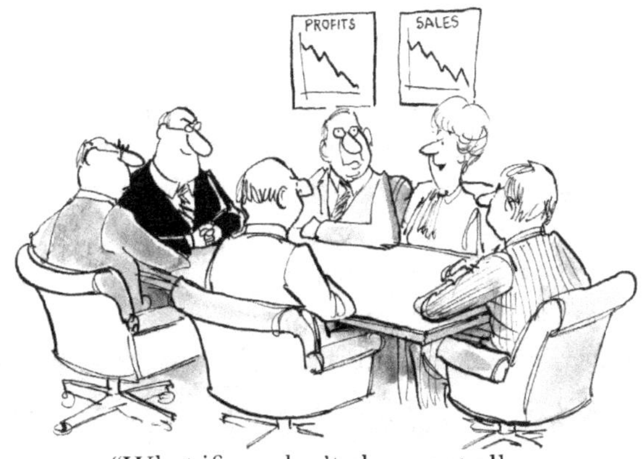

"What if we don't change at all ...
and something magical just happens?"

Information

It is time to select a **Fast** path to recovery suitable to your specific needs. No matter whatever path it is, you are aiming at the same target: reducing your insulin resistance, eliminating the internal fat from inside and around your vital organs, and allowing your liver and pancreas to do the natural work for you.

In the end, your fat will literally dissolve into thin air. When your fat is lost, 84% of it leaves your body through exhaling and only 16% is metabolized into water (H_2O) that's excreted via the sweat glands and waste. And as this happens, your vital organs are freed — unshackled of fat — to function normally without the enemy of "insulin resistance" sabotaging your efforts.

As soon as your vital organs are free from fat and your cells are once again able to readily accept insulin's magic, the heavy load is removed, and they can do the job they were genetically conceived to do, including the management of your glucose intake.

The key is to confidently select a fasting routine that you know you can do. As I mentioned earlier, not everyone can do the 24-hour fast. You may want to begin on the 16-hour program and progress to 24 hours of non-eating, or somewhere between 12 and 24 hours of fasting once you realize it's not nearly as scary as you're now thinking. Or you may be super-pumped and dive straight into a 5 or 7-day fast or the 24-hour routine. It's completely up to you and your doctor.

Remember, this is a process you will embrace in one way, shape or form for the rest of your life.

We'll go from toughest to easiest. Ready? Let's go!

7-Day (or any Consecutive-Day) Fasting

- Fasting week (days): Pick a day and time in the next few weeks to stop eating for seven consecutive days, 24 hours a day, total of 168 hours.

- Your #1 goal is to drink plenty of fluids and stay hydrated. If on medications, you also must monitor your blood-sugar levels in conjunction with your doctor's advice and assistance.

- Allowable fluids include water, tea, coffee (with a tad of milk permitted), and broths (bone or vegetable with added sea salt or Himalayan salt). For all of the foregoing, add no sweetening agents of any kind, including artificial sweeteners.

- Though you must maintain hydration, do not overdo it. Just maintain normal fluid intake (8 glasses, 125 ml each, per day), which is itself a goodly amount of liquid.

- Follow this same fasting program for any number of days from 2 to 7.

24-Hour Fast x 2 or 3 Days per Week (Intermittent Fasting)

- Fasting days: Start by selecting two or three days from the week, Monday to Wednesday, Monday-Wednesday-Friday, Tuesday-Thursday, for example, ideally the same days each week for consistency and pattern. Exactly when you will start and stop, such as dinner-to-dinner, breakfast-to-breakfast, or lunch-to-lunch, depends on your schedule and trial and error.

- Non-fasting days: These are the other four or five days of the week when you eat. Ideally, when eating on these days, choose low-carb, low-GI foods for your shopping basket (carbs are not essential to the human diet), as described in more detail in the next chapter, limit yourself to a maximum of three meals per day (evenly spaced), eliminate all snacks, and always use a smaller portion or portion plate as a guide when eating.

- Body Clock: On Non-fasting days when you do eat, be sure to honor your body's natural 12-hour body clock. This means you should eat only during the day when your body naturally desires to metabolize food most efficiently.

16-Hour Fast x 2 or 3 Days per Week (Intermittent Fasting)

- Fasting days: Initially select two days per week to stop eating for a continuous period of 16 hours. 7 pm one day, until 11 am the next, for example, is a common selection, as it overlaps with your sleep period and thus makes it natural and comparatively easy.

- Non-fasting days: Again, these are the other four or five days of the week when you eat. Again, eat only low-carb, low-GI foods, limit yourself to a maximum of three meals per day, shun snacks, and eat smaller portions.

- Query: If you can stop eating during the day, then why not for the 24-hour fast since you'll be sleeping (ideally) for six to eight of those hours anyway?

- Suggestion: Increase the number of fasting days as you go, after your body and mind adjust to the new regimen and you get into the flow.

12-Hour Intermittent Fasting with Low-GI Foods

- Under this option, you only eat during the body's 12-hour body clock, preferably daytime hours between about 6 am to 6 pm or 7 am to 7 pm.

- Ideally, do this every day of the week. If you can't, try every other day and go from there.

For all options, when not fasting, i.e., on days and during periods of time when you are eating, be sure to observe the following guidelines:

- ☞ Drastically restrict intake of carbs. If you must eat carbs, select only low-carb foods for your shopping basket, to complement veggies and low-GI fruits.

- ☞ Eat no more than 3 meals per day, and for each meal, eat smaller portions (using a smaller portion plate if that helps).

- ☞ NEVER snack between meals (if tempted, first drink a large glass of water to hydrate you and see if that fills you up — often it will, and you will no longer be hungry).

- ☞ Honor your body clock by eating only during the allotted period ideally during daylight hours and never outside a 12-hour period.

*How will you know when your selected **Fast** option is working?*

It will be self-evident. You will shed pounds and your blood glucose readings will be progressively reduced. With weight loss, your insulin resistance and diabetes will improve instantly, and, within a matter of weeks, you will see measurable improvement as validated by your new A1c, HbA 1c, or Hb 1c hemoglobin reading.

These readings are used interchangeably and all measure, in lay terms, the level of sugar or glucose in your blood. More specifically, it measures the average blood glucose over three months. Your goal is to achieve an A1C 7%, which may be reported as eAG: 154mg/dl. Through following the guidelines in this book, many people will take control of their diabetes in two to three months (or less).

Once you have achieved your goal, be guided by your blood-sugar readings and weight. If you see your weight creeping back up and your blood-sugar readings climbing, then another **Fasting** may be in order. And maybe some high-GI carbs have insinuated themselves back into your regular diet, in which case they need to be tossed in the rubbish and not ordered or purchased to begin with.

Which is not to say that you should stop enjoying life. Just the opposite. You can still eat freely at your friend's wedding or on special occasions. You can still have a "naughty" meal once in a while and you can still enjoy a couple of glasses of wine, beer, or alcoholic concoction at select social gatherings. Just remember to keep it to a minimum and get straight back on target the next day.

Before I conclude the chapter on **Fasting**, I want to add one parting caution. **Fasting** isn't for everyone. Fasting is not recommended for children under the age of 18, anyone with a low BMI, anyone who is frail or recovering from illness, any women who are pregnant or breastfeeding.

And of course, as always, if you have any significant illness such as epilepsy or Parkinson's, or you are currently taking blood pressure tablets or diabetic medications of any kind, be sure to first discuss fasting with your physician.

Action

Select a *Fasting* routine that best fits your sensibilities and lifestyle. Write it down here and include the reasons for your particular selection over the others:

____

____

____

____

Write here and in your calendar the *Fasting* days and times you have selected for your personal *Fast* option. Be specific as to what date and time you will start and finish for each week and then each week of the month going forward:

____

____

____

____

Start a **Healthy Living Diary** to record the food, recipes, portion sizes, and times you eat. This will enable you to tweak your choices to find what works best for you.

Put your **Healthy Living Calendar** in plain sight, such as on your fridge, kitchen counter, or bedroom wall, and your giant marker gleefully cross off each milestone day as you progress, beginning with Finished Book: **X**!

Chapter 8
YOUR SMART FOOD CHOICES

"Dis-moi ce que tu manges, je te dirai ce que tu es."
("Tell me what you eat, and I will tell you what you are.")

— Anthelme Brillat-Savarin

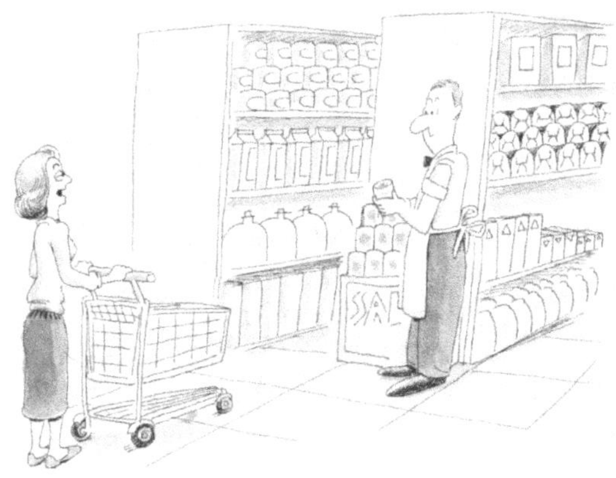

"In what aisle are the
'won't immediately kill you' foods?"

Information

Eating the right foods is crucial to your **Fast Diabetes Solution**. Making smart choices like grass-fed meat and fresh, organic vegetables, including acidic and bitter foods, is best.

By eliminating processed food, fast food, fried foods, food additives, processed sugar, table salt, HFCS, sweet and salty snacks, refined starches (whole wheat, bread, flour, pasta and rice), high fructose fruits (in large quantities) and fruit juices, bad oils, and all bad carbs as much and as often as possible, you will literally be extending your own healthy life.

If it's in a box, or frozen, or has a long shelf life, be especially aware of the ingredients. Indeed, make reading and understanding food ingredients — what you're putting into your gut — your new hobby (even obsession)!

So, let's start right here with a review of Carbs, Protein, Fats, Bitter Foods, Foods with Enzymes, Acids, Anti-inflammatory Foods, Anthocyanins, the Okinawa Phenomenon, Lemons, Spices, Starch, and Alcohol — because all have a major impact on your dietary health, including your prospects for contracting or reversing type 2 diabetes:

Carbohydrates

As we know, your total food GI is critical: substituting high-GI foods for low-GI foods and finding the right balance between them and the right amounts is the goal. This means substituting high-GI Carbs with low-GI Carbs (basmati rice instead of jasmine rice, sourdough bread over white or whole wheat bread, and so on), and consuming smaller portions of most things.

Protein

Lean, preferably free-range and grass-fed red meat (with increased omega-3 fatty acids), fish (with an eye toward avoiding exposure to mercury), pasture-raised or free-range chicken and eggs, legumes, nuts, seeds, and the like — all keep your GI low when consumed in moderation. Eliminate all processed meats, such as fast food hamburgers, fried chicken patties, and many packaged luncheon meats, as they all are toxic to the bowel and a major cause of inflammation and insulin resistance.

Fats

Omega-3 fatty acids are good for you and are anti-inflammatory. These include: fish like salmon, tuna, mackerel, anchovies, and sardines; nuts and seeds like walnuts, chia seeds, and flaxseeds; egg yolks from fresh, free-range chickens; and grass-fed meats.

Also good for you are (1) monounsaturated fats, which come from vegetables and natural oils and nuts, such as olives, olive oil, nut butters, avocado, cashews, walnuts, peanuts, almonds, brazil nuts, pistachios, pecans, peanuts, and canola, and (2) saturated fats, which come from coconut oil, butter, and ghee. All provide healthy, natural fats and do not contribute to inflammation.

Gut-Friendly Foods

There are two types of foods: Prebiotic and Probiotic.

Prebiotic. Good prebiotic, gut-friendly foods are those providing dietary fibers as a food source for probiotic bacteria in the gut, encouraging the proliferation of a healthy gut microbiome environment. These most commonly include apples, bananas, blueberries, leeks, onions, garlic, legumes, chia seeds, beans, artichokes, and asparagus, root vegetables like carrots and beets, and cabbage.

Probiotic: Good probiotic, gut-friendly foods are usually fermented foods packed with beneficial bacteria, including homemade pickles, sauerkraut, kimchi, homemade yogurt with active yeast (ideally eaten 1–2 tablespoons with meals), and kombucha.

Bitter Foods

Bitterness can be very good to you. Bitter foods encourage bile flow in the liver and gallbladder, thereby aiding digestion. These include endives, rocket, dandelion, bitter melon, and artichokes.

Acids

Acidic foods tend to lower blood glucose and aid digestion — lemon juice, vinegar, apple cider, balsamic, and the like. As little as one tablespoon of vinegar added to a meal has been found to lower the blood glucose response to that meal by 30%. Similar results have been found for lemon juice.

Foods with Enzymes

The best known of these are tropical fruits (available in most stores), are pineapple, mango, and papaya. Organic wax honey is preferred as a sweetener. All aid in digestion and when consumed in moderation, contribute to a healthy diet. However, all of these should be avoided or highly restricted during your *Fasting* recovery stages due to their carb and fructose content.

Anti-Inflammatory Foods

Olive oil, fish (salmon, mackerel, tuna, sardines), tomatoes, leafy green vegetables (spinach, kale, collard greens), almonds, walnuts, flaxseed, chia seeds, hemp seeds, and fruits like blueberries, strawberries, cherries and oranges — all are high in omega-3 fatty acids and/or deemed anti-inflammatory. Same caution for fruits, however, during **Fasting** recovery stage.

Anthocyanins

The potent anti-inflammatory and antioxidant qualities of anthocyanins are often found in vegetables and fruits colored blue, purple, and red. Examples are blueberries, blackberries, cranberries, strawberries, apples, peaches, dry grape seeds, red wine, cacao, radicchio, purple sweet potatoes, purple cauliflower and asparagus, red cabbage, aubergines (eggplant), plums, beetroot, figs, and blackcurrant. High quantities of anthocyanins with their protective flavonoids have been shown to improve eyesight, slow dementia, and improve cardiovascular conditions as well as positively address diabetes. Blueberries, in particular, have been shown to improve blood glucose levels. However, the fruit with one of the highest levels of anthocyanins is the blackcurrant. Again, restrict anything sweet and high in fructose during your fasting recovery stage.

Okinawa Phenomenon

Interestingly, on Okinawa Island, Japan, living to over 100 years of age and still enjoying an active life is common. Investigations into the vitality and longevity of Okinawans reveals that their diet includes very high levels of anthocyanins, which they find mainly in the purple sweet potato which is indigenous to the island. Of course, other aspects of Okinawan life, such as respect for elders and a relaxed pace of life may also be significant — reminding us that good health is holistic in all respects.

Lemons

Carbohydrates are found in lots of fruits, but fruits have wildly varying GIs, so attention must be paid to the selection you make. Generally, the more acidic the fruit, the lower the GI. Lemons, for example, have little or no carbs and therefore negligible GI, whereas cherries or blueberries have much higher GIs of around 60. Which is not to say we wish to condemn you to a life of lemons, though it would not be all bad, as these fruits are also chocked full of valuable nutrients and thus provide valuable additions to any diet. Being packed with anti-oxidants and low in fructose they also mop up the free radicals known to be involved in many illnesses. In particular, when added to meals, lemons slow down glucose absorption with considerable favorable results.

Spices

As will be discussed in much more depth later in the book, as we have devoted a whole chapter to them, spices are a phenomenal source of health. Spices like cinnamon, turmeric (which is also anti-inflammatory), *Gymnema sylvestre*, sumac, cloves, sage, curry leaves, garlic, turmeric, cayenne, fenugreek, ginseng, ginger, rosemary, oregano, marjoram — all contribute to lower blood glucose.

Starch

Starch is a complex carbohydrate found in many foods such as grains, starchy vegetables, legumes, and beans. Resistant starches are particularly difficult to break down and thus stay in the gut much longer, offering several health benefits. Not only do they provide a food source for gut bacteria and encourage a healthy gut microbiome, they reduce the absorption of toxic compounds which would otherwise increase inflammation. As resistant starches, they also make us feel fuller longer (putting them high on the satiety index) and slow down the absorption of food from the gut, so as not to cause a rapid increase in blood glucose. The more highly processed a food, by the way, the lower the level of resistant starch present. To increase your consumption of resistant starches, you need to increase your consumption of whole foods. Modern diets for Westerners typically offer a tenth of the level of resistant starch compared to those of people living in underdeveloped countries; so making a dietary adjustment is usually necessary.

Alcohol

To achieve maximum weight loss, alcohol should be avoided during your *Fast* **Diabetes Recovery** period and moderated for life. Of course, it is important that you allow yourself the freedom to enjoy life — and if that means tossing back the occasional pint while watching football, or enjoying a glass of wine with your loved one or friends, that's fine. We are not trying to turn you into a teetotaller, but there are certain drinks which score much higher on the carbo-insulin scale.

From better to worse, in terms of carbs, are champagne (surprisingly enough, only one gram of carb per serving, red wine (at two grams per serving), white wine (three grams), and beer (13 grams, hence "the beer gut" phenomenon). Hard alcohol, on the other hand, varies much from zero carbs to off the charts, depending on what it is and what it is mixed with.

Whiskey, dry martini, brandy, tequila, vodka, vodka and soda water — all weigh in at zero carbs. Ramp it up for a Bloody Mary (7 grams of carbs per serving), Margarita (8), Cosmopolitan (13), White Russian (17), Vodka & Orange Juice (28), and Rum & Coke (39). Notice how the carbs jump with the addition of fruit juice and soda pop.

The **Fasting** option you chose needs to be realistic, enjoyable and blend as seamlessly as possible with your life and lifestyle. Otherwise, it will become another restrictive diet forcing you to fall off the healthy food wagon and never get back on.

The point that bears repeating about alcohol is that, from a healthy lifestyle perspective, it must always be consumed in moderation. It has little nutritional value, and because the body does not store it, it is the first nutrient used for energy. And while the body is busy burning up alcohol, it isn't burning your stored fat accumulation. As a result, alcohol makes you fat and getting fat defeats your goal of reversing diabetes and living a happy, healthy, diabetes-free life.

In the end, what is most important is making a permanent lifestyle change that improves and maintains good health, while keeping diabetes away forever.

Action

Make a solid list of the good, healthy foods you like, based on the information provided above or other reliable sources:

Low-GI Carbs

Protein

Fats

Bitter Foods

Suzanne Ridley

Foods with Enzymes

Acids

Anti-Inflammatory Foods

Chapter 9
YOUR SHOPPING BASKET

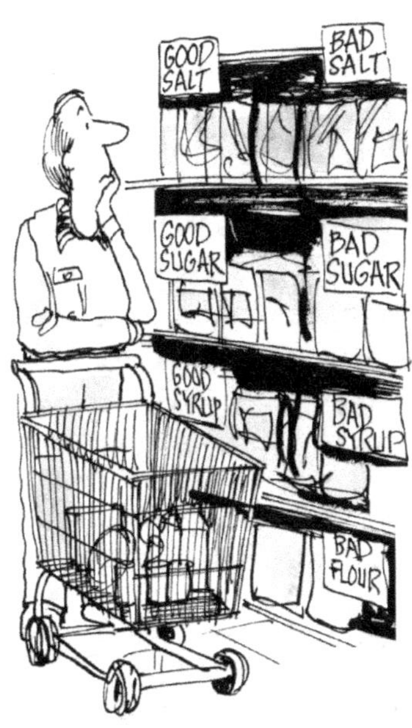

Information

You've now made a list of healthy foods that you like. In this chapter, we focus on your Shopping Basket — what to include and what to avoid. This is the crux of the eating side of the new you (start eating healthy right away, regardless of when you start *Fasting*.

During your recovery phase (before you have reversed your diabetes) it is important that you avoid foods that negatively impact the diabetic condition, such as: bread, rice, pasta, high-fructose fruits and high-GI vegetables. After the recovery phase, you can enjoy these foods in moderation.

The key to assembling a healthy shopping basket is to include a wide range of diverse and healthy foods, with an eye towards everything that's low in GI, low in carbs, low in fructose, fresh, wholesome, organic vegetables and nuts is a good place to start. Mix in fresh fish, free-range, organic red meat and chicken, and you'll enjoy some amazing meals. In fact, once you master the art of healthy eating, you'll look back and wonder why you ever did it any other way.

*Although we advocate "fresh is best", it is not always a practical way to live. Just be sure when eating canned or frozen foods that you are looking closely at the ingredients with a focus on avoiding preservatives, sugars, salt and any ingredient name you can't pronounce — they're bound not to be natural or healthy.

Your Recovery Phase Shopping Basket

Vegetables and Fruit

Fill your shopping basket with a variety of healthy, tasty and colorful foods — here are some to get you started:

- o Broccoli, Brussels sprouts, bok choy, cabbage, cauliflower
- o Aubergine (eggplant)

- o Tomato
- o Avocado
- o Olives
- o Lemon, lime, grapefruit
- o Mushrooms
- o Courgette (zucchini)
- o Peas, green beans
- o Lettuce (especially bitter lettuce such as radicchio, arugula/rocket hold the best nutritional value)
- o Spinach, kale
- o Artichoke
- o Asparagus
- o Celery
- o Carrot
- o Bitter melon
- o Onion (red onions are high in chromium and antioxidants)
- o Pumpkin
- o Bell peppers (capsicum)
- o Chilies
- o Cucumber
- o Garlic

Note: During your recovery phase avoid most fruits due to fructose content (stick to the few listed above) and steer clear of the high-GI veggies such as: potatoes, parsnips, beetroot, and yams.

Suzanne Ridley

Meats

- o Grass-fed beef, lamb, pork (grass-fed protein is higher in omega-3 fatty acids)
- o Free-range chicken, turkey, duck

Seafood

- o Fish (deep-sea fish, in particular, which is higher in omega-3 fatty acids)
- o Shrimp (prawns), lobster, crab
- o Oysters, clams, scallops, octopus, squid

Eggs

- o Free-range eggs (good source of B-vitamins, including biotin– B_7)

Milk (unsweetened)

(Note: Make sure your choices, where applicable, are of the full-fat variety)

- o Cow's milk
- o Goat's milk
- o Soy milk
- o Almond milk, macadamia milk

Yogurts – (full-fat)

- o Plain and unsweetened

Cheese – (full-fat)

(The longer a cheese is aged, the lower the carbohydrate content)

- o Cheddar

- o Blue cheese
- o Goat's cheese
- o Mozzarella
- o Parmesan
- o Brie

Saturated Fats

- o Butter
- o Cream
- o Ghee
- o Coconut oil

Monounsaturated Fats

- o Olive oil
- o Avocado
- o Olives

Vinegars

- o Apple cider
- o Balsamic
- o Red wine vinegar

Spices

- o Turmeric
- o Cinnamon
- o Sumac
- o Cumin
- o Paprika
- o Fenugreek

- o Ginger
- o Rosemary
- o Oregano
- o Marjoram
- o Pepper

Miscellaneous Items

- o Coconut flour
- o Almond meal (flour)
- o Himalayan salt or sea salt (use sparingly)
- o Cacao (powerful antioxidant)
- o Coffee
- o Tea
- o Stevia (herb – organic sweetener)

After Your Recovery Phase, You Can Add These to Your Shopping Basket to Enjoy in Moderation

- Seeds – chia, sesame, pumpkin, flaxseeds, sunflower, quinoa

- Nuts (unsalted) – brazil nuts, walnuts, almonds, cashews, peanuts, macadamias, pecans, pistachios, hazelnuts

- Fruits – blueberries, blackberries, strawberries, blackcurrants, goji berries, pomegranate, kiwi fruit, apple, oranges, banana (technically a herb) — limit high-fructose fruits to small amounts occasionally

- Legumes – lentils, chickpeas, hummus, black-eyed beans, red kidney beans, butter beans, cannellini beans, soya beans, mung beans — small portions, see potion plate below (resistant starches are highly nutritious)

- Grains – basmati rice, brown rice, steel cut oats, buckwheat, amaranth, millet — small portions see portion plate below

- Cheese – cottage cheese, ricotta cheese, cream cheese

- Starch vegetables – sweet potato, beetroot, yam, and potato — limit your consumption to small amounts occasionally, see portion plate below

- Meats – bacon, ham (off the bone), salami, cured and smoked meats to be consumed in small amounts occasionally

- Dark chocolate (aim for 85% cocoa with correspondingly less sugar)

- Organic honey in small amounts (high fructose) — limit your consumption to small amounts occasionally

- Bread – sourdough and multi-grain — limit to the occasional single slice

- Pasta – small quantities — see portion plate below

*Tip for cooking rice and pasta — after cooking, cool the rice or pasta in the fridge overnight to either be reheated or added cold to a dish. This changes the food structure to a more resistant starch which lowers the GI response.

Portion Plate

When you choose to eat grains or starchy foods use this portion plate as a guide.

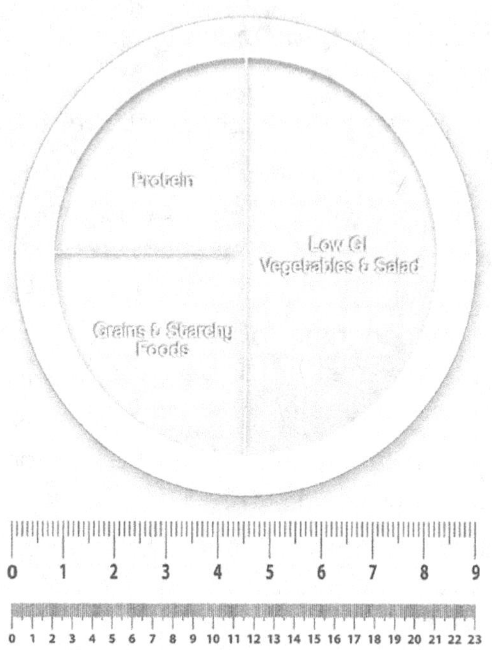

Action

Write down your new Healthy Shopping List, including a healthy mix and balance of all varieties discussed:

Once you're done, jump into your car, go to the farmer's market if you have one, or the store with the freshest, organic veggies.

Don't forget to buy a big garbage bag when you are at the supermarket. Because when you get back home, it will be time to fill it up with all the unhealthy foods that you no longer want in your life. You will never need these foods again. These foods are the old you. Note how good you feel as you throw the "rubbish foods" away and fill your shelves with wonderful, tasty alternatives. And just for fun, itemize all the items you are tossing. In several months, you can look back and see just how far you've come.

Need more space?

Chapter 10
HERBS, SPICES & MINERALS

"All those spices and herbs in your spice rack can do more than provide calorie-free, natural flavorings to enhance and make food delicious. They're also an incredible source of antioxidants and help rev up your metabolism and improve your health at the same time."

– Suzanne Somers

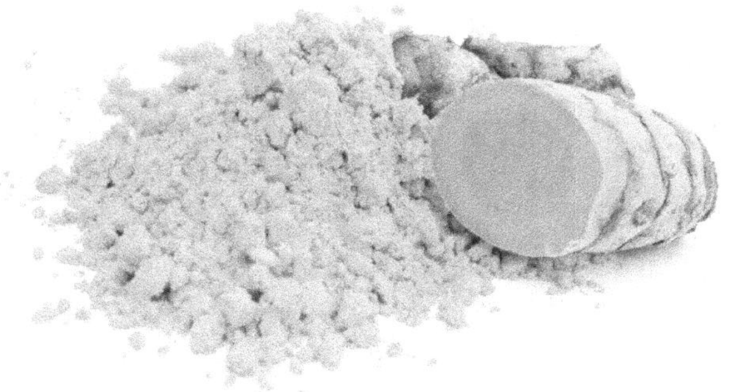

Information

Spices are part of human history. In 3000 BC, India's southwestern port of Kerala became known as the "Spice Garden of India." The Silk Road — on which spices like cinnamon, pepper, ginger, and turmeric were transported — became the arterial trade route between Europe and Asia. And when Columbus in 1492 sailed the ocean blue in search of the "Spice Garden of India," instead he found what became known as the Americas.

Before gold and the creation of money, spices like peppercorn could be used to pay rent. Throughout the 16th century, Spain and Portugal played tug-a-war over cloves. In Indonesia, the British and the Dutch fought over nutmeg, with hostilities ceasing upon the exchange of the tiny island of Run (going to the Dutch), in return for the then-worthless land that became Manhattan (going to the British).

Though spices historically served commerce as much as health, today most scientists agree that spices provide profound health benefits, ranging from combating inflammation to improving digestion and helping conquer type 2 diabetes. Wouldn't it be amazing if Mother Earth offered us a natural, safe, accessible, and tasty alternative to conventional pharmaceutical drugs with their long lists of often-debilitating negative side-effects?

Brilliantly, there are: Herbs, Spices, and Minerals.

Despite their complex nature, herbs and spices don't have a single property like pharmaceutical drugs. Many are profoundly complex, providing multiple beneficial attributes that can easily be worked into your *Fast* **Diabetes-Free Lifestyle**. Whether you are able to *Fast* reverse your diabetes or not, controlling your diabetes is a life-long journey, and the right mix of herbs, spices, and minerals is essential to maintaining a healthy you.

In this chapter, we have curated a list of herbs, minerals, and spices which will help you reverse and cure your diabetes. Some qualify as super-spices, while others deliver important but less vibrant benefits. I hope you find them as exciting, tasty and beneficial as I do.

The Super-Spice: Turmeric, Turmeric Root Extract & Curcumin

Turmeric is one of the most powerful nutritional supplements in existence. Many studies establish its beneficial effects over your brain and your body. Rich in curcuminoids, this is the ingredient that makes it a strong antioxidant and powerful anti-inflammatory agent, as well as giving curry its rich, yellow color.

The curcuminoids in turmeric deliver a host of positive health effects, including lowering blood glucose and blood lipids and reducing inflammation. These qualities, combined with its antioxidant effect, provide wonderful protection against cardiovascular and many other chronic diseases.

A leading study took place over nine months in 2012, in which all subjects had been diagnosed with pre-diabetes before the study began. Over that nine months, one group was given curcumin and the other group a placebo. The result was spectacular: not one person taking curcumin progressed to a diagnosis of type 2 diabetes, while 16.4% of the placebo group did. Other benefits from curcumin and negligible side-effects were also noted.

When thinking of turmeric, however, remember that most studies establishing turmeric extract's positive impact on type 2 diabetes entail intense dosages of curcumin, usually in excess of 1 gram per day. Eating enough turmeric spice in food to achieve this level of consumption would be very difficult.

And even if you poured it onto every meal, problems remain: curcumin absorbs poorly into the bloodstream. To aid in the difficult absorption process, I strongly recommend that you consume curcumin with black pepper, which contains piperine. Piperine is the natural substance which enhances by 2,000% the body's ability to absorb curcumin.

Taken the right way, including heating it up and dashing on the pepper, here is a list of highly beneficial qualities of turmeric.

- It has powerful medicinal properties
- It's a natural inflammatory
- It contains high antioxidant properties
- It's been linked to improved brain function and lower risk of brain disease
- It lowers the risk of heart disease
- Due to reduced inflammation, it is a potential cancer prohibitive
- Arthritis responds to curcumin supplement
- It quells depression
- It may delay aging and fight other age-related chronic diseases

The Sugar Destroyer Spice: The Ayurvedic Herb, *Gymnema Sylvestre*

Those who battle a sweet tooth will benefit from the super-herb *Gymnema sylvestre*. Having a chemical configuration mimicking sugar, it fills the sugar receptors in your taste buds, blocking your ability to taste sweetness.

Native to India and Africa, it can be found indigenously as a climbing vine. For centuries the crushed leaves of *Gymnema sylvestre* were used to create the herb gymnema, which is part of India's Ayurvedic medicine tradition. In Hindi, the root word "gumar" literally means "destroyer of sugar."

Research also suggests that this herb compromises your intestine's capacity to absorb glucose thereby reducing your blood sugar (or blood glucose) levels. It does so by curbing the binding of carbohydrates to the receptors in the intestines.

Recently, a clinical trial proved that taking a certain dose of gymnema daily (400 mg), enjoyed a significant success in controlling hyperglycemia — through significant reductions in blood sugar, hemoglobin A1c, and glycosylated plasma protein levels. After 18 months, participants in this study were able to reduce their drug dosages and five of the participants regained normal blood glucose levels using this herb alone as a good supplement.

As a result of these studies and many, many more, its prescriptive uses today include general treatment of type 2 diabetes, metabolic syndrome, weight loss, appetite suppressant and even use as a diuretic.

Suzanne Ridley

A Mineral – Chromium Picolinate

Chromium is an integral mineral found in the earth's voluminous seawater and crust. In animals, it is found mainly in organ meats and whole grains. As trivalent chromium, look for it to be contained in most foods in trace amounts and often included in nutrient supplements.

Its interest in health — and in addressing diabetes in particular — harks back to the 1950s, when it was deemed to substantially lower plasma glucose levels in diabetic mice. Following a dip in attention, in the 1970s interest in chromium renewed when its consumption by diabetics led scientists to conclude that it constitutes an essential nutrient necessary for carbohydrate metabolism.

Further study has since found that diets rich in refined carbohydrates are low in chromium. Accordingly, scientists have concluded that chromium is clearly involved as a glucose tolerance factor, invigorating the efficacy of insulin by increasing the number of insulin receptors.

Chromium comes in several forms, the most effective being chromium chloride, which has been shown to improve blood-sugar readings when consumed either before or after eating. As the UK's official site on diabetes states: "Chromium is of interest to people with diabetes as it has been suggested that Chromium Picolinate could be particularly suitable for lowering blood-sugar levels."

The Vitamin – Biotin

Biotin is a member of the B-vitamin group. It is found in egg yolks, whole grains, liver, and vegetables, and also is a co-factor in many enzyme systems.

Scientists have found that a combination of *chromium(III) picolinate* and *biotin* improve blood-sugar control, thus limiting the need for medications in diabetics and the obese. One study published in *Diabetes Metabolism Research Review* reported that taking a daily supplement of 600 mcg of chromium(III) picolinate, combined with 2 mg of biotin, brought about a 6% drop in fasting blood-sugar levels.

Study co-author Dr. Ira Goldfine of the University of California, San Francisco, commented: "Our findings show that chromium plus biotin can improve blood glucose and reduce HbAlc in patients with type 2 diabetes, especially in those who have the poorest control... These effects could result in significant reductions in diabetes-related complications."

Thus, the belief is that biotin enhances the established benefits provided by chromium(III) in managing diabetic symptoms.

The Common Table Spice – Pepper

Pepper is a 4,000-year-old spice, all varieties coming from the vine *Piper nigrum*. The different kinds — green, black, white — depend on age of ripening and how they are processed. Picked before ripening are green peppercorns. Picked after ripening are black peppercorns. Both are then sun-dried, which darkens the skin. If you remove the skin, usually early in the process when it is easier, you have white peppercorns.

Much research confirms the positive health effects of pepper. It works wonders on arthritis, inflammation, and even pain perception. Studies suggest it addresses type 2 diabetes as well, working as a strong antioxidant. It also serves as a valuable catalyst or delivery mechanism, improving the body's healthy absorption of nutrients from food and food supplements.

Scientists have taken a very close look at piperine, which is the active phenolic compound found in extractions of black pepper. They have learned that even in low doses piperine inhibits interleukin 6, which is pro-inflammatory, and MMP13, a gene tied to arthritis and metastasis. It also was found to minimize prostaglandin, a pro-inflammatory hormone, and substantially curb joint inflammation in mice.

A Rising Spice Star – Sumac

The tangy berries, roots, and leaves of sumac (*Rhus glabra L.*) have been providing folk remedies for centuries. Dried and ground, the edible *Rhus* species delivers a flavorful lemony taste to meat and vegetable dishes; it has shown scientific promise as a strong antioxidant, control agent for glycemia and bad cholesterol; and it is a valuable contributor to improved cardiovascular health.

In research, it provided glycemic control and lowered cholesterol levels. A double-blind, placebo-controlled study published in the *Iranian Journal of Pharmaceutical Research* in fall 2014 reported an interesting finding: type 2 diabetic patients might be able to reap a wide range of health benefits by adding sumac to their diets.

At the end of the three-month trial period, patients who had been taking three grams of ground *Rhus coriaria L.* (Sicilian sumac) daily enjoyed significantly lower levels of blood glucose, Apolipoprotein B (the so-called *bad cholesterol*), and HbAlc (the type of hemoglobin that is measured to identify the average plasma glucose concentration over prolonged periods of time).

At the end of the trial, the sumac group also showed increased levels of TAC (total antioxidant capacity) and apoAl (a component of the so-called *good cholesterol*). In short, the health benefits of Sumac are supported by good science.

Another Super-Spice: Cinnamon

It is hard to beat cinnamon as a delicious and healthy addition to your daily diet. Revered as a food flavoring and medicinal spice since time immemorial, it lowers blood-sugar levels, reduces risks of heart disease, and provides a host of other benefits.

As there are different types, picking the best one to ingest is important. It is better to use Ceylon, or "true" cinnamon, because not all cinnamon is created equally. The cassia variety contains significant amounts of a compound called coumarin, which is believed to be harmful in large doses. All cinnamon should have health benefits, but cassia may cause problems in large doses due to the coumarin content. Ceylon ("true" cinnamon) is much better in this regard, and studies show that it is much lower in coumarin than the cassia variety. Unfortunately, most cinnamon found in supermarkets are of the cheaper cassia variety.

That aside, through hundreds of studies modern science has validated what Ayurvedic medicine, holistic healers and millions of people have known for ages. You can Google and read about all the beneficial qualities of cinnamon, but you're liable to be busy for the rest of the year. For a synthesis, see the study released by the *Annals of Family Medicine* that seeks to make sense of all the previous cinnamon studies as pertains just to diabetes. It examines 10 different studies undertaken with a total of 540 people, all suffering from type 2 diabetes. Though doses varied between studies, daily intake ranged from 120 mg to 3g. The result: taking cinnamon around meal times is a definite winner in tackling diabetes.

At the end of the day, cinnamon is one of the most delicious and healthiest spices on the planet. It can lower blood-sugar levels, reduce heart disease risk factors, and provide a plethora of other impressive health benefits. Just make sure to get Ceylon cinnamon, or stick to small doses if you're using the cassia variety.

Magnesium – a Mineral

The blood of type 2 diabetics is known to be low in magnesium, so it makes sense that increased doses of magnesium will improve diabetes. One such study, published in the *American Journal of Clinical Nutrition*, found that daily Magnesium supplements activate glucose transport, improve the behavior of hormone regulators, and improve overall oxidative glucose metabolism. Another, undertaken by researchers at the Harvard School of Public Health in January 2004, reported a significant correlation between magnesium intake and risk of type 2 diabetes. Their report was the result of two large-scale, long-term studies following over 170,000 health professionals and evaluating diet and its impact on disease: *The Nurses' Health Study* and the *Health Professionals' Follow-Up Study*.

Conclusion

The list of herbs, spices, and minerals goes on and on and so could I. At the end of the day, by controlling your blood glucose through smart food choices that include taking herbal and nutritional supplements, you'll make huge strides toward the permanent resolution of your type 2 diabetes. Fasting, eating a healthy diet of the right low-GI foods, reducing your portion sizes, eating only during your body clock window, and taking herbal supplements — from a dietary point-of-view, all will help you achieve a healthy and happy life that is diabetes-free.

Action

Detail any and all spices, nutrients, and supplements you have taken over the years. Also, describe any impact on your health that they seem to have brought:

____

____

____

____

Do the same for any current spices, nutrients, and supplements you are taking:

____

____

____

____

____

____

Chapter 11
PHYSICAL ACTIVITY & EXERCISE

"Time is the most valuable commodity we have because there are only two guarantees in life:
1. At some point in time you are going to die
2. If you don't go after what you really want in life you'll die before you get it
So stop waiting and start moving."

— Patrick Ridley

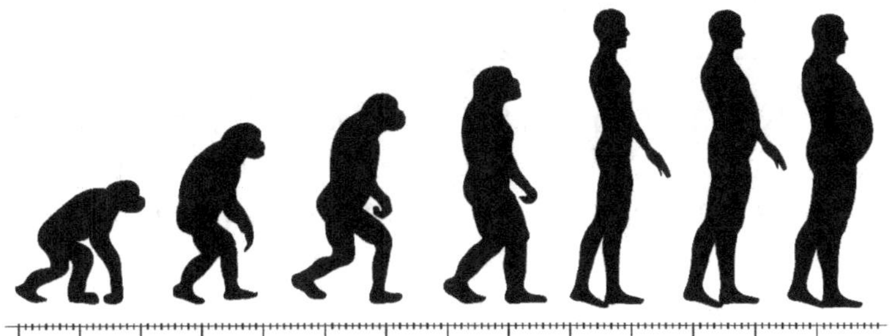

Information

In the quest for health and happiness, physical activity — good, old-fashioned daily exercise — plays an important role. The much-vaunted Mayo Clinic lists these benefits from regularly exercising your body:

- ⊃ Controlling your weight by burning fat.

- ⊃ Decreasing your risk of heart disease by preventing high blood pressure, stimulating good cholesterol, and reducing nasty triglycerides.

- ⊃ Elevating your emotional well-being through stimulation of brain chemicals such as endorphins with a resultant boost in confidence and self-esteem from feeling and looking good.

- ⊃ Increasing energy and vitality, muscular strength, and endurance via the delivery of oxygen and essential nutrients throughout the body.

- ⊃ Ensuring better and deeper sleep as the body seeks naturally to re-set itself, rest and recover from exertion.

- ⊃ Stimulating and boosting your sex life, through greater energy and higher production of hormones that excite sexual arousal, release, and satisfaction.

- ⊃ And last but not least, it's fun, and when you laugh, your views of everything tend to improve, including especially your optimism.

Now, if these benefits alone were not enough, and if physical activity — exercise — is important to health, then working the body is crucial to battling type 2 diabetes.

For starters, two new studies, one on mice and another on obese humans, reveal definitive evidence that exercise changes the composition of gut microbes independent of diet or antibiotic use. We have explained in a previous chapter the significance of having a healthy gut for improved mood, weight control, warding off Alzheimer's and combating type 2 diabetes.

Exercise also boosts the millions of cells in your body to become more sensitive to insulin and more receptive to its natural wonders when you are exercising and exerting yourself physically. Studies show that good fitness enables your cells to work far more efficiently and effectively in removing unwanted glucose from your blood. During exercise, a mechanism totally separate from insulin itself takes on the glucose challenge.

Those currently taking diabetes-related pills know that an energized exercise routine, if followed consistently, lowers your blood glucose as evidenced by measurably improved A1c. And as your A1c test results improve, your doctor cuts back your pill dosage or reduces your required insulin intake. The foundation to exercise curbing diabetes begins here.

But what kind of physical activity — what kind of exercise — will best assist you to accomplish your current mission to reverse type 2 diabetes?

To that question, I have an answer, and it fits brilliantly with **Fasting**. The answer is high-intensity interval training, known more popularly as HIIT.

HIIT

HIIT is the exercise routine whereby high-intensity exercise is alternated with rest or low-intensity exercise. Sounds much more complicated than it is. Think of it generally as sprinting then resting, sprinting then resting, sprinting then resting. The sprinting can take the form of anything — running and walking, fast treadmill and slow treadmill, quick weight reps then resting.

To better explain it, let's tap into something you know. Most of you are familiar with aerobic exercise, which today is often called cardio. Jogging for long periods of time around the park, running on the treadmill until you're drenched in sweat, or riding the unicycle or exercise bike in the health club while reading a magazine or surfing the net — these are all aerobic forms of exercise and standard fare in today's world.

We call this type of physical activity aerobic for the way it impacts your body. Aerobic means "relating to, involving, or requiring free oxygen," so as to meet energy demands during exertion and impact your aerobic metabolism. The notion is that the longer you go, the more calories and thus the more fat you will burn. Many workout machines track this for you as you go, displaying the results on a monitor with blinking dots and dashes.

Though HIIT includes an aerobic component, it also has something else, and that something else is what makes me select HIIT as the best exercise method for improving your health, losing weight and assisting you to reverse type 2 diabetes. High-intensity interval training is primarily an anaerobic exercise. Not aerobic, but anaerobic. Only a few letters, but they make a world of difference. Anaerobic exercise means literally "without oxygen." So, while aerobic exercise is "with oxygen," anaerobic exercise is without it.

What then is the advantage of anaerobic exercise over aerobic exercise in the battle against diabetes?

"In research, HIIT has been shown to burn adipose tissue more efficiently than low-intensity [aerobic] exercise up to 50% more efficiently." Being anaerobic in nature, HIIT hits you hard in the first 10 to 15 seconds of your work out, exhausting your phosphate pool, and then provides the energy for all of your efforts up to one minute before involving glycolysis and lactic acid. It thus provides a benefit over normal cardio by combining anaerobic and aerobic results that burn more fat.

With fat as our target, let's cut to the chase. HIIT is the best exercise model for tackling diabetes because it is the best exercise routine for reducing fat quickly, effectively, and over the long term. And unlike aerobic exercises, whose fat-burning qualities wane quickly after cooling off, HIIT's anaerobic side burns fat for 24 to 48 hours after our workout is through. It's a double-whammy.

And there's more. HIIT accomplishes multiple goals at once. It not only causes substantial fat loss, it also improves both aerobic and anaerobic endurance with fast results in a short period of time. "A study at Laval University in Quebec, Canada, found HIIT cardio helped trainees lose nine times more fat than those who trained in the traditional way with moderate speed for 20–60 minutes." The result is that HIIT's impact on the body is unparalleled so as to offer a superior method for battling diabetes.

Why?

Because the overall goal is reduction of body fat, and HIIT does it best.

Tabata

There are of course many ways to approach high-intensity interval training. Enter Dr. Izumi Tabata, the dean of Ritsumeikan University Graduate School of Sport and Health Science in Japan. His name has become famous in the sports and health world by virtue of the so-called "Tabata Protocol." The "Tabata Protocol" applies HIIT uniquely based upon a series of studies.

Dr. Tabata took two groups of Japanese athletes — speed skaters — and put them through comparative training programs for six weeks. One group engaged high-intensity, "Tabata-style" training of 20 seconds on, ten seconds off, for a period of four minutes. The control group engaged in moderate to intense continual exercise — a typical aerobic workout — for one hour. Both groups exercised five days a week, taking two for rest, for the entire six-week period.

The result was a dramatic and substantial comparative reduction in body fat for the "Tabata-style" workout, despite it only being four minutes in duration for five days a week. The reason is that the spiked intensity of the workouts caused the body's metabolism to jump, and raised the heart rate rapidly.

This, in turn, burned fat during the exercise period and caused the body's metabolism to continue to burn fat for another 24–48 hours, something aerobics cannot do.

The Benefits of Tabata

With workouts as short as four minutes, Tabata training can achieve a host of amazing benefits:

- ✪ It increases testosterone levels (testosterone being the ultimate muscle-building and fat-burning hormone)

- ✪ It improves muscular oxidative capabilities of your mitochondria (this is the power-house of the muscular cells)

- ✪ It provides an upsurge of GLUT 4 quantities (GLUT 4 is the insulin-regulated glucose transporter)

- ✪ It enlarges cell dimensions of the myofibrillar within the muscle tissues.

Obscure jargon, I know, but the point is that a Tabata exercise model increases human growth hormone levels by about 350% while burning fat and building muscle. Insulin sensitivity is also boosted via Tabata, enabling glucose to be taken from the bloodstream and absorbed into the muscles rather than stored as unwanted body fat. Coupled with this reduction in your fat storage potential is an increase in carbohydrate metabolism post workout, for 24–48 hours, which helps shift excess body fat to muscle.

The Tabata Workout

Perhaps all of this sounds a bit abstract, so let's get to the nitty-gritty. The Tabata workout is simply an exercise routine. Certain exercises are more suitable than others, but let's start with running. You can do it outside, but you don't have to — because you can just as effectively run in place.

With Tabata, you're going to work out for four minutes, cycling through intervals of 20:10. For twenty seconds, run in place as fast as you can without stressing your joints, then drop your pace and jog slowly in place for ten seconds. Repeat this routine twice a minute for four minutes. Sounds easy, but I promise you it will feel like a long four minutes.

Running is just one option among many. Squats, crunches, toe-touches, lunges (front and side), butt kicks, knee lifts, arm circles, trunk twists, and side bends all work more or less as effectively as running, and all can be done from the privacy of your home. If you have access to a health club or gym, then you also have choices like the treadmill, unicycle, rowing, barbells, weights, and such.

The key is to go as fast as you can when in sprint mode. Of course, as with any strenuous exercise, always warm up first with modest jogging in place and stretching of the muscles and limbs. After your warm up, immediately begin your exercise routine. If you are out of shape or haven't worked out in a while, start with one exercise and go for four minutes. If you're able, switch to a new exercise and continue on with that exercise for another four minutes. If you still feel able, do it one more time with a new exercise for a total of 12 minutes, which brings you even with the Tabata test group.

Do this five days a week for six weeks and see how you feel. I guarantee you that you will burn fat, shed pounds, be thinner, look better, and feel healthier or happier for this reason alone. But here's the catch: you're not doing HIIT or Tabata in isolation. You are combining it with **Fasting** and after the **Fasting** recovery period is over, you're combining Tabata with a healthy diet for the rest of your life.

But that's not all. To reverse and cure your diabetes, you're combining Tabata, regular physical activity, **Fasting**, and a healthy diet — with restful sleep and stress control.

Action

Write out by day all of the physical activity you currently do over a typical week, including workouts, regular walking or jogging, and leisure (walking the dog, going on hikes, and so forth):

Monday:

Tuesday:

Wednesday:

Thursday:

Friday:

Suzanne Ridley

Saturday:

____

Sunday:

____

Write down your new commitment:

Monday:

____

____

Tuesday:

____

____

Wednesday:

____

____

Thursday:

____

____

Friday:

____

____

Saturday:

____

____

Sunday:

____

____

With your new exercise program in place, write down what is motivating you to become fit, healthy, and diabetes-free? For example: "I am becoming fit and healthy to have more quality time with my children and grandchildren."

1)
____

2)
____

3)
____

4)
____

5)
____

Then post your motivations on stick-ems everywhere you can think of — at home, at work, in your car, everywhere. There they will serve as a daily reminder and motivator to stay on target.

Chapter 12
SLEEP, STRESS CONTROL & MEDITATION

"Professor: We have our final exam tomorrow."
"Student: What should we do to prepare?"
"Professor: Get a good night's rest."

— Anonymous Ethics Professor

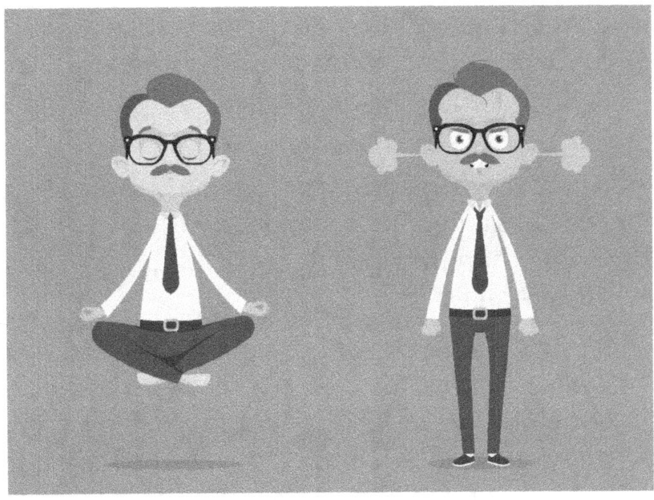

Information

Sleep and stress reduction are two factors commonly overlooked when it comes to type 2 diabetes. However, both play a significant role in preventing its onset, helping to reverse and cure it, and improving your overall health.

Sleep

I found a quote that really captures the benefits of sleep. Alyssa Sparacino, Editor for *Shape & Fitness* online, said: "Sleep makes you feel better, but its importance goes way beyond just boosting your mood or banishing under-eye circles. Adequate sleep is a key part of a healthy lifestyle, and can benefit your heart, weight, and mind."

The Benefits of Sleep

Separate and apart from feeling rested, a good, sound, and deep sleep provides a host of wonderful human benefits. Here are but a few:

➡ It reduces inflammation, which is linked to diabetes, cardiovascular disease, stroke, arthritis, high blood pressure, and premature aging.

➡ It improves memory, attention, creativity, and mental acuity. As we all know, there is nothing worse than facing a challenging day with a bad night's sleep.

➡ It aids the body in burning fat and losing weight. One University of Chicago study concluded that, of the weight lost by a group of dieters, 56% more fat was burned from those who slept well, and that sleep deprivation causes hunger hormones to intensify.

➡ It helps to manage stress by enabling our minds and bodies to re-set and recharge themselves. Sleep deprivation, on the other hand, causes new stress and aggravates existing stress, as it interferes with muscle repair, memory consolidation, and acuity.

➡ It contributes to and worsens depression. Anxiety, worry, pessimism, and a sense of hopelessness — all can flow from chronic sleep deprivation and sleep disorders.

Sleep, Diabetes, and other Ailments

With respect to diabetes in particular, research establishes that poor sleep habits lead to higher blood glucose levels and increased insulin resistance, which as we know are antithetical to reversing diabetic symptoms.

In one study published in Diabetes Care, researchers assessed the sleep patterns of 40 people with type 2 diabetes over six nights, following them for insomnia, sleep apnea and snoring. They also took blood samples to analyze insulin and glucose levels.

The study revealed that diabetics who were also poor sleepers suffered 23% higher levels of blood glucose in the morning, as well as 48% higher levels of blood insulin. For insulin resistance, these figures meant that poor sleepers with diabetes had 82% higher insulin resistance than normal sleepers with diabetes.

Kristen Knutson, lead author on the study, commented: "People who have a hard time controlling their blood glucose levels have a greater risk of complications. They have a reduced quality of life. And they have a reduced life expectancy." Serious words, to be sure.

Eve Van Cauter, co-author of the study, added: "This suggests that improving sleep quality in diabetics would have a similar beneficial effect as the most commonly used anti-diabetes drugs."

As many of you may already know, diabetics are generally known to have worse sleep patterns than non-diabetics, leading some experts to identify chronic sleep problems as creating a potential risk for developing diabetes in the first place.

Indeed, studies unequivocally demonstrate that untreated sleep problems, especially sleep apnea, can increase the risk of obesity, insulin resistance, and type 2 diabetes. Night-shift workers with abnormal sleep patterns — including sleep apnea — also report these problems.

Sleep apnea is a common disorder whereby a person's breathing is interrupted during sleep. Individuals with sleep apnea often move out of deep sleep and into light sleep when their breathing pauses or becomes shallow. This results in poor sleep quality that leads to sleepiness or exhaustion during the day.

Unfortunately, many people aren't aware of their symptoms and aren't diagnosed. If you think you might be one such person, be sure to inform your doctor. It may well extend your life. More information about sleep problems is available from the National Heart, Lung, and Blood Institute at:

www.nhlbi.nih.gov/health/resources/sleep

Furthermore, obesity correlates to both diabetes and sleep apnea, making both more likely to occur. This is due to the impact of sleep deprivation on hunger hormones. In this connection, I was blown away by the results of Sharad Taheri's Bristol University study, which concluded that sleep-deprived individuals have 15% more ghrelin, which is the hormone that tells us to eat more, and 16% less leptin, which tells us to stop eating.

In the modern age of computers, monitors and digital screens, Dan Pardi's studies at Stanford University and Leiden University are also telling. Because sleep is so tied to light, many people are having their sleep disrupted by the omnipresence of blue light emitted by mobile phones, tablets, laptops, digital screens and even modern-day lights. This impacts the body's production of melatonin, the hormone that helps us sleep, and as a result, the body's circadian rhythm is so out of whack that it becomes confused.

Pardi's view is that sleep disruption can even impact our gut flora, making the usually-diligent flora inefficient at their work in digestion and nutrient absorption. He also opines that chronic lack of sleep not only impacts restfulness and alertness during waking hours, but contributes to obesity, metabolic syndrome, weight gain, fat accumulation, type 2 diabetes, and even cancer.

Experts tend to agree that each and every one of us should routinely get between six and eight hours of deep, undisrupted sleep. It is my strong view that doing so will help you reverse your diabetes or not contract it in the first place.

Tips for a Better Sleep

For those with sleep issues, Dr. Robert Buist of the International Academy of Nutrition offers a host of suggestions on how to get a better night's sleep. These include:

- ☞ Taking a warm bath at night accompanied by gentle music;

- ☞ Writing out tomorrow's tasks to avoid worry while sleeping;

- ☞ Turning off all light sources (TV, computer screens);

- ☞ Exercise earlier in the day, thus creating a higher need to sleep and repair;

- ☞ Eliminate excess caffeine and alcohol consumption, and;

- ☞ Go to sleep at the same time each night after a warm lemon and honey drink.

There must be many more as well, and I would love for you to share them with me and other readers. Let's turn now to the subject of *Stress.*

Stress

You know it well. Pressure, time deadlines, overwork, mental and physical demands of the modern world — all cause debilitating stress, if not managed. Management is the key, because the stressors are not going away. They are part and parcel of life.

Stress often originates in the world around you. Your boss, your spouse or partner, your children, your neighbors, life changes, litigation, a politician or politics in general, the latest negative media story, deadlines. But the external stimulants are just the beginning. Stress starts there and then goes inside you. In other words, you internalize it.

Inside you, the little devils causing stress are aptly-named "stress hormones." These hormones, that include both adrenaline and cortisol, mobilize stored energy in the form of glucose and fatty acids. This energy mobilization is part of your "fight or flight" response and is useful to prepare individuals to deal with stressors.

For individuals without diabetes, these energy sources can be quickly utilized. However, for those of you with diabetes, the presence of significant insulin insensitivity causes the newly-released glucose to build up in the bloodstream. Over time this leads to chronic inflammation and many of the ills which it delivers: diabetes, metabolism malfunction, obesity, and hypertension.

Many of you may be experiencing illness of some sort, blaming it and only it for your nagging headache, inability to sleep soundly, and poor work or personal performance. But the real culprit may be chronic stress, stress that is accumulating over time, and stress in combination with the illness. Psychological stress makes your physical stress worse. And vice-versa. It's an endless circle and should be promptly addressed.

To see if you are suffering from ongoing stress, take the adrenal fatigue quiz online at:

www.intacad.com.au/2017/02/recognising-the-
adrenally-fatigued-patient-2/

... as suggested by the International Academy of Nutrition.

Stress & Diabetes

Stress makes things worse for diabetics. Studies confirm that it raises your blood-sugar levels and exacerbates many unhealthy habits which further worsen your diabetes, like smoking, consuming excess alcohol, avoiding exercise and healthy activity, and eating too much of the wrong thing at the wrong times.

Stress & Obesity

Stress triggers production of the hormone cortisol. Cortisol is a well-known contributor to belly fat. Unfortunately, belly fat or fat that's layered around your vital organs and abdomen, pose a greater risk to health than other stores of body fat.

Managing Stress

There are lots of things that you can do to manage stress, all of which will help to reverse and cure your diabetes over the long run. These vary from the profound, such as making a complete lifestyle change as urged by this book, to the simple and nuanced, such as putting a good book at your bedside and actually reading it after taking a warm bath in a room lighted only by tea candles.

Try all or any combination of the following to reduce, manage and control your stress:

o   Be active and exercise, even if it means taking the dog for a walk or going for a peaceful walk around the nearest park.

o   Find time and ways to relax, such as meditation, yoga, deep breathing, bathing in candlelight, getting a massage, doing tai chi, devouring a good book.

o   Be positive and try to have a sense of humor. For example, make the first thing you say in the morning a happy one. And remember, a bad joke told is better than none ventured at all. Create a morning routine that puts you in a calm and happy state that you can continue through the rest of the day.

o   Get out. Mix, socialize, go places and see people. Rarely will your entire outing be without a fun surprise or interesting tidbit that puts you in a good mood.

o   Find a hobby. Everyone has a hobby in them. Gardening, bird-watching, hiking, fishing, surfing, art, reading, acting, playing guitar, flying drones, drawing, painting, building models — all bring great joy to your life while keeping you focused and active.

o   Unwind. Make sure you give yourself some time to unwind and relax. If you are like me, it is very easy to make this a low priority; but when you consider the effects mentioned above, you now know you must treat this aspect of your new lifestyle change with high importance in terms of your health and both reversing and curing diabetes.

Finding the balance of infinite options that work in your life is the challenge and the goal. Start with a few; mix, match, and experiment; then expand or retract to enhance your results. At all times you are your own study. A study of one. So look in the mirror, reflect on your thoughts, and try to see yourself from a distance. Harmony should be your end result.

When Help Is Needed

Sometimes your condition continues despite taking positive steps at stress reduction and maintenance. In these cases, see your doctor, consider a professional counselor or therapist, and look for other potential causes. Locating the source of your stress and finding tools to cope with it are your motivations.

Lowering Your Blood Pressure

Studies suggest that diabetics with controlled blood pressure within the normal range are 30% less likely to suffer from diabetes-related complications, including stress, heart attack, and strokes, when compared to their hypertensive counterparts. These studies suggest that normalizing your blood pressure alone will improve your life expectancy and quality of life more than lowering your blood glucose levels. How's that for a shocker.

Mindfulness and Meditation

Mindfulness Meditation has been shown to help reduce your HbAl. This is the measurement, if you'll recall, of your average blood glucose levels over the prior weeks and months. Mindfulness meditation has been shown to increase glycemic control and subsequently reduce the chances of having hyperglycemic episodes, leading to a reduction of the mental distress associated with diabetes management.

In one study, a team of researchers led by Dr. Debra Rosenzweig tasked participants to complete a mindfulness course for eight weeks, along with maintaining a diary of the exercise and diet regimes. Within a month, HbA 1c and blood pressure measures were significantly reduced in the mindfulness participants as compared to others.

The beauty of mindfulness meditation is its simplicity. You simply concentrate inwardly with your breath, focusing on the physical sensations in your body or even that quiet space in your mind, usually when sitting cross-legged with your back erect (or whatever is comfortable). You don't have to master the full lotus position to reap the benefits of meditation.

Start with something achievable at the beginning. Doing an hour of sitting meditation every day may be too much. If you can manage this at the beginning, then go for it; otherwise, try just 10 to 15 minutes in the morning, and another 10 to 15 minutes at lunch or during your afternoon break.

Here are two different mindfulness meditations:

The Calm Breath Technique

1) Go to a quiet place where you won't be interrupted. Sit with your legs crossed and back straight if you can or do so with the aid of a chair.

2) Close your eyes and bring your awareness to your breath. Take some deep breaths and really let go and relax with every exhalation.

3) After several deep breaths, allow your breathing to become calm and natural. Note the sensations of your breathing within your body. Pay close attention to the rise and fall of your chest and the sensations of the air passing through your nostrils onto your upper lip. Remain in this quiet place with complete focus. If your mind starts to wonder, or you find yourself thinking about tasks or worries, accept them and then without a care permit them to float away like a feather in the wind. Then bring your attention back to your calm natural breath and relax, going deeper and deeper as your body harmonizes with your breathing.

4) When you feel it's time to return to the outer world, take a final moment and make a conscious decision to stay calm and relaxed by saying to yourself: "I am relaxed and calm and I will remain in this state throughout the day. I will be alert, refreshed and energized. I will be calm, focused, and capable of dealing with anything that comes my way

The Body Sweep Technique

1) Go to a quiet place where you will be not be interrupted. Sit with your legs crossed and back straight if you can or do so with the aid of a chair.

2) Close your eyes and bring your awareness to the top of your head. Let your focus stay there for a while and notice all the different sensations that

arise. You may feel a sense of warmth, a tingling or tickling, a pulsating sensation, a compression, a lightness or the reverse, a heaviness. Whatever you can feel place your awareness over it. If you cannot identify any sensations, just accept it and relax, leaving your awareness at the top of your head.

3) Move your focus onto your face, starting with the forehead and being aware of any sensation that may come or fade away. Move your attention slowly down over your eyebrows and onto your eyelids. Stay relaxed with calm and natural breaths, allowing your awareness to move into your nose then spread to your cheeks and ears, down your neck and onto the tops of your shoulders. Spend some time in each place, feeling the sensations.

4) Continue the process from your shoulders down to your arms, hands, and fingers.

5) After reaching your fingers, bring your attention to your chest, moving from there down to your stomach and then further down to your groin.

6) From your groin bring your awareness back up to the top of your back and then move slowly down to the small of your back and from there to your buttocks.

7) After your buttocks, place your attention over your hips and then thighs, moving to your knees and then down to your lower legs.

8) Lastly, move your focus over your ankles and then down to your feet and toes.

9) Once you have completed a full body scan, go
   back to the top of the head and do a slow sweep
   over all of your body in the same sequence, being
   aware of any sensations you can feel. You can do
   this as many times as you wish.

Action

Make a list of all the stressors in your life, rating them
on a scale of 1 to 10, 10 being the most stressful, and 1
being the least:

❶

❷

❸

❹

❺

❻

❼

❽

❾

❿

Identity the ways, applying the techniques discussed in the book that you will now address and manage these stressors as part of your new Diabetes-Free Lifestyle Plan:

Start your stress-free life now by taking 5 to 10 minutes to go through one of the mindfulness exercises described in this chapter. After you finish, note how you felt before and afterwards.

PART III: PUTTING IT ALL TOGETHER – YOUR PLAN

Chapter 13
YOUR *FAST* DIABETES-FREE LIFESTYLE PLAN

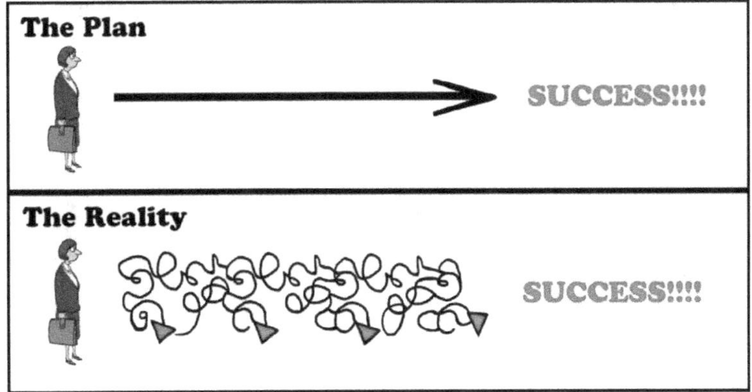

The Plan

The ~~End~~ Beginning

You have come to the end of the book but the beginning of your new diabetes-free life.

What next?

What are you going to do right now to reverse and cure your diabetes and realize your dreams of LIVING a healthy and happy life?

We'll help you do it, but we must do it together.

Ready?

Okay, pick up your pen again and start filling in the blanks below. If you get tired, take a break, drink some water, go for an invigorating walk, and then get back to it.

Before you know it, you will be done.

Your *Fast* Diabetes-Free Lifestyle Plan

Fasting – select a ***Fast*** option and make any relevant notes:

7-Day Fasting

Start date and time:

____

Notes on Drinks and Broth:

____

2–3 Day Fasting

Start date and time:

____

Days of the week:

____

Notes on Drinks and Broth:

Shopping List for Non-Fasting Days:

Recipes for Non-Fasting Days:

24-Hour Fasting

Start date and time:

Start date each week for balance of the month:

Shopping List for Non-Fasting Days:

Recipes for Non-Fasting Days:

Diet

Make a shopping list built around healthy menu options for all of your daily meals:

Healthy, Low-Carb, Low-Sugar Diet

Shopping Cart for Eating Days, including Food, Spices, and Minerals (when you are not Fasting):

Monday

Tuesday

Wednesday

____

____

Thursday

____

____

Friday

____

____

Saturday

____

____

Sunday

____

____

Menu Options for Eating Days, including Herbs, Spices, and Minerals (when you are not Fasting)

All Days – eating timeframe: _______________________________
(For example, 8:00 am–6:00 pm)

Monday

1st Meal:
____

2nd Meal:
____

3rd Meal:
____

Suzanne Ridley

Tuesday

1st Meal:

2nd Meal:

3rd Meal:

Wednesday

1st Meal:

2nd Meal:

3rd Meal:

Thursday

1st Meal:

2nd Meal:

3rd Meal:

Friday

1st Meal

2nd Meal:

3rd Meal:

Saturday

1st Meal:

2nd Meal:

3rd Meal:

Sunday

1st Meal:

2nd Meal:

3rd Meal:

Physical Activities & Exercise

(HIIT, Tabata training, yoga, city and nature walks, enjoying life, the arts, ecstatic dancing, music, films, and so on, as your time permits)

Monday

Tuesday

Wednesday

Thursday

Friday

Saturday

Sunday

Suzanne Ridley

Stress Management

(Mindfulness Meditation, Yoga, Spiritual Time)

Monday

Tuesday

Wednesday

Thursday

Friday

Saturday

Sunday

Sleep

(A good night's sleep of 6–8 hours — indicate a regular bedtime consistent with your family needs and lifestyle)

Monday: ___________   Friday: ___________

Tuesday: ___________   Saturday: ___________

Wednesday: ___________   Sunday: ___________

Thursday: ___________

There you go. How simple was that? Now you have your own, personalized *Fasting* **and Diabetes-Free Lifestyle Plan**. If you need any help or inspiration along the way, we offer you a couple of options:

- ✪ You can join and engage in our online *Fast* **Diabetes-Free Lifestyle Community** on Facebook — where you can ask us any question you may have.

- ✪ You can join our **Diabetes Recovery Program** — contact support@puranutrients.com for more information or visit www.puranutrients.com

Success starts with a small first step which you have already taken by reading this book.

It follows by creating and implementing your *Fast* **Diabetes-Free Lifestyle Plan**.

Of course, if one combination doesn't work, or if you have a false start, or stumble along the way. Simply dust yourself off and start over again.

The famous inventor Thomas Edison "failed" 1,000 times in his pursuit to create the light bulb. When a reporter asked, "How did it feel to fail 1,000 times?" Edison replied, "I didn't fail 1,000 times. The light bulb was an invention with 1,000 steps."

To give up is when you truly fail. In trying times remember your motivators in life: your children, grandchildren, retirement, quality of life and just the sheer joy of feeling healthy and free of diabetes — and you will feel your enthusiasm returning in full force.

No matter which way you do it, your life sentence to type 2 diabetes, heart disease, and expensive medication is over as you've known it (or, at the very least, has taken a major turn for the good). Reach up and give yourself a hearty pat on the back. Please share your success story on our *Fast* **Diabetes-Free Solution Facebook Group**!

Final Tips to Remember on Your Journey

As you get ready to begin the next phase of your life, here are some final thoughts:

- Make sure you have read this entire book and answer the questions after each chapter.

- Discuss with your doctor your suitability for fasting, any need for medication adjustment, and any weight-loss considerations — especially decreased pill dosages as your blood glucose level drops (and it will!).

- Clean out your cupboard, fridge, and freezer of any and all items that don't meet your new healthy food criteria: healthy, fresh, organic (where possible), low-carb, and low-GI.

- Eat healthy three times per day and only during your optimal body clock.

- Buy a portion plate so that you can easily serve up the correct portions of each food type (use smaller plates and bowls when dishing out your meals) NO SECOND HELPINGS!

- Purchase a Blood Glucose reader to monitor your blood glucose levels. Take and record regular readings in your diary and follow your amazing progress.

☞ Begin your new physical activity and exercise regime today.

☞ Set aside time for meditation every day and twice daily when possible.

☞ Commit yourself to a life as stress-free as you can realistically make it.

☞ Get a good night's sleep every night with a standard bedtime and eliminate blue light two hours before retiring.

☞ Join "The *Fast* Diabetes Solution" Facebook community for extra support and guidance.

☞ Complete a daily Diabetes-Free Diary, noting any mentionable things that happened during the day and your feelings about how you are doing on your path to recovery.

☞ Periodically check in with your doctor on your progress.

☞ For a huge confidence boost go back and look at the answers you gave early on in the book, noting how far you've come.

☞ For an even bigger confidence boost, pull up the photo you took when you started and compare it to the new, you!!!

☞ Enjoy your new, diabetes-free life, and remember to let us know when you have done it!!!

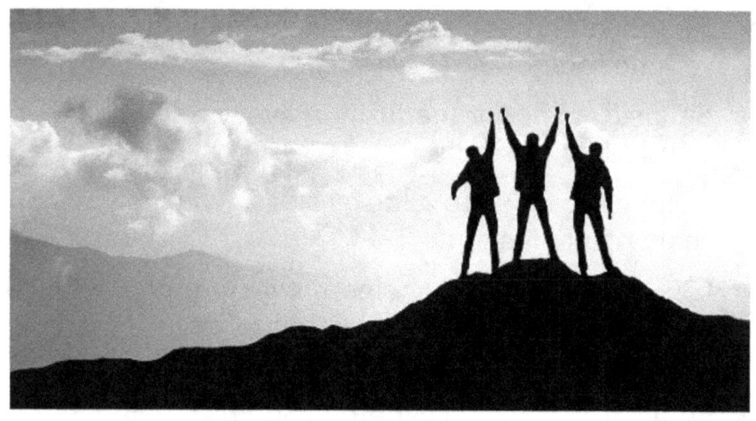

Thrive, live and be happy with your new *Fast* Diabetes-Free Lifestyle.

"Success is nothing more than a few simple disciplines, practiced every day."

— Jim Rohn

Recommended Reading

Grain Brain by Dr. David Perlmutter

Low GI Diet Handbook by Professor Jennie Brand-Miller

The Gut Health Diet Plan by Christine Bailey

The Obesity Code by Dr. Jason Fung

What the Fat by Professor Grant Schofield, Dr. Caryn Zinn, and Craig Rodger

Why We Sleep by Professor Matthew Walker

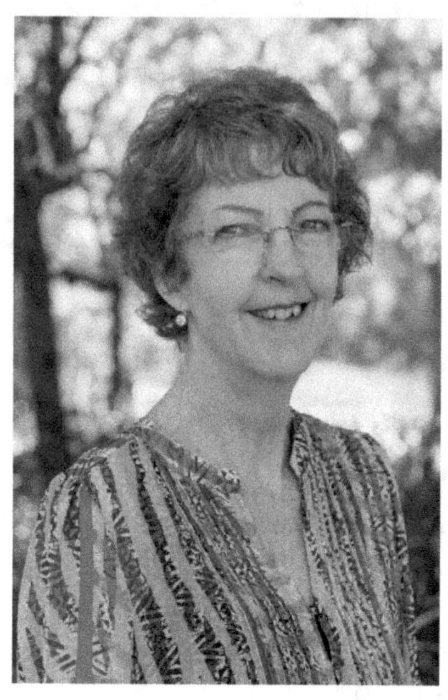

Suzanne Ridley is a pharmacist with over 40 years' experience and holds qualifications in clinical nutrition and medical herbalism. Suzanne has combined her knowledge of pharmaceutical drugs, nutrition, and herbs to tackle the biggest pandemic of modern times — type 2 diabetes. She is the Principal Health Specialist and Co-founder of Pura Nutrients, a health and well-being company specializing in the treatment of type 2 diabetes and health optimization for healthy, happy living. Suzanne lives in the Blue Mountains west of Sydney, Australia, with her husband, Ray.

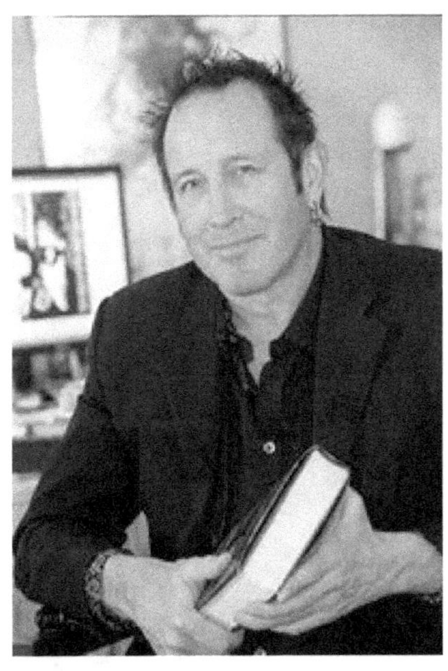

Steve Eggleston is a law school Valedictorian, former law professor, lecturer, and colorful American trial lawyer who left home at age 16 and worked his way through school. Over the years, his clients and adversaries have included con men, swindlers, greedy families, drug addicts, big oil & big tobacco, Fortune 100 companies, entertainment giants, writers, and Grammy-winners. His debut fiction thriller, *CONFLICTED*, received high critical acclaim, and he is published in both fiction and non-fiction as a writer, co-writer, and ghostwriter in genres as diverse as health and inspirational memoirs. He lives with his family in magical Somerset, England.